MENTAL HEALTH CARE IN THE WORLD OF WORK

Mental Health Care

This research demonstration was supported in part by Grant no. RO-1-MH-14890 from the National Institute of Mental Health and Grant no. RD-1453-G from the Rehabilitation Services Administration, both of the Department of Health, Education, and Welfare, Washington, D.C.

in the World of Work

By HYMAN J. WEINER

SHEILA H. AKABAS

JOHN J. SOMMER

Foreword by Bertram S. Brown, M.D.

Director, National Institute of Mental Health
United States Department of Health, Education and Welfare

ASSOCIATION PRESS

NEW YORK

MENTAL HEALTH CARE IN THE WORLD OF WORK

Copyright © 1973 by Association Press

Association Press, 291 Broadway, New York, N.Y. 10007

International Standard Book Number: 0-8096-1863-X
Library of Congress Catalog Card Number: 73–8653

LIBRARY OF CONGRESS CATALOGING IN PUBLICATION DATA

Weiner, Hyman J
  Mental health care in the world of work.

  Bibliography: p.
  1. Industrial psychiatry. I. Akabas, Sheila H.,
1931–   joint author. II. Sommer, John J., 1924–
joint author. III. Title. [DNLM: 1. Mental health
services. 2. Occupational health services. WA495
W423m 1973]
RC967.W43   362.8'5   73–8653
ISBN 0–8096–1863–X

Printed in the United States of America

To our unfailingly patient
and understanding spouses—
Shirley, Aaron and Svea

Contents

Foreword

The 1966 edition of the *Random House Dictionary of the English Language* defines work as follows:

WORK: Exertion or effort directed to produce or accomplish something. Synonym: drudgery, toil, labor. Antonym: play, rest.

Spanning centuries of human history, one finds in the Bible a similar definition in Genesis 3:19: "In the sweat of your face you shall eat bread."

Over the years, the subject of work has been examined from social, economic, and political points of view. Work has also been examined in a variety of moral, religious, and philosophical frameworks. For example, work provides a sense of reality according to Freud. Elton Mayo believes work is a bind for the community. For Marx, its function is economic.

More recently, scholars have been concerned with the meaning of work and its social purposes. Elliot Jacques summarizes the relationship between work and self-esteem in this way:

. . . working for a living is one of the basic activities in a man's life. By forcing him to come to grips with his environment, with the actuality of his personal capacity—to exercise judgment, to achieve concrete and specific results, gives him a continuous account of his correspondence between outside reality and the inner perception of that reality, as well as an account of the accuracy of his appraisal of himself. . . . In short, a man's work does not satisfy his material needs alone. In a very deep sense, it gives him a measure of his sanity.

The National Advisory Commission on Civil Disorders, addressing the problem of poverty and unemployment more concretely states:

> The capacity to obtain and hold a "good job" is the traditional test of participation in American society. Steady employment with adequate compensation provides both purchasing power and social status. It develops the capabilities, confidence and self-esteem an individual needs to be a responsible citizen and provides a basis for stable family life.

These brief and diverse quotations illustrate that work plays a pervasive and powerful role in our lives. The work environment today is a crucial focus of adult life. It is the source of the means of economic survival, life satisfactions, and, inevitably, of stresses. Technological developments are substantially altering the nature of work and presenting new challenges which both employees and management must master. In addition, the emergence of large complex work organizations is making new demands on people for expertise in dealing with the social aspects of the work setting. Along with these technological and social changes comes a high potential for psychological stress.

Work has an extremely important role in our lives—in economic, social, psychological and physical terms. How many of us, for example, spend more non-sleep time at work than at home? Individuals express their personal and family problems, their fears, insecurities, frustrations, loneliness, and alienation at work and through their work. The highest executive, the union leader, and the worker on the assembly line all experience and must deal with the tragic conditions that result from the emotional trials of coworkers, colleagues and supervisors. Emotional disturbances and mental illness can touch all of us. Therefore, in humanistic, economic and social terms, the world of work is a basic concern of the field of mental health.

Mental illness is without a doubt the nation's costliest health problem and constitutes an enormous drain on the country's energies and resources. Consider the following facts:

1. Accidents, low productivity, and high personnel turnover are concrete industrial problems significantly related to mental health and mental illness.

2. Emotional problems are responsible for approximately 20 to 30 per cent of employee absenteeism.

3. Personal factors cause 80 to 90 per cent of industrial accidents.

4. It is estimated that from 15 to 30 per cent of the work force are seriously handicapped by emotional problems. This may be only a guess, but evidence shows that about a quarter of any large work force is in serious need of help for some kind of psychological and social trouble.

5. At least 65 and possibly as much as 80 per cent of the people who are fired by industry are dropped from their jobs because of personal rather than technical factors.

6. Although exact dimensions are unknown, there are considerable data which suggest that drug abuse and addiction is emerging as a serious and major problem in many work settings.

7. At least a $15 billion loss to the economy occurs annually as a result of alcoholism and alcohol abuse. Of this total, lost work time in industry, government and the military, accounts for $10 billion. Health and welfare services provided to alcoholics and their families cost $2 billion. An estimated 3 to 3.5 billion dollars may be attributed to property damage, medical expenses, increased insurance costs, and wage losses.

Mental-health professionals have contributed ably and thoughtfully to the vast literature on *work*. However, until very recently, few have sought to use the work setting as a vehicle through which to find the worker in trouble and to help that worker stay on the job. This book presents some of the important and innovative aspects of the work-mental health relationship. The dedicated and highly competent researchers associated with this study demonstrate that it is productive to harness the various components of the work environment in support of a work rehabilitation program geared to keeping blue-collar workers with emotional problems on the job. When this study was carried out in the mid-1960's the mental health needs and problems of blue-collar and industrial workers were unnoticed and unsung. In addition, mental-health services to these workers and their families were negligible. Where they were available, the world of work, its relevance and its role in treatment were unnoticed and unused in most cases.

The study team of this research-demonstration study pioneered in their effort to combine the resources of the unions and management, along with their ancillary organizations, such as the Health Center, the insurance company, and community mental health programs. This enabled men and women with emotional problems or mental illness to continue their employment in the "world of work." This was neither a minor challenge nor a small accomplishment. The book notes the trials and tribulations, successes and failures. We are indebted to the researchers for their honest, forthright and thoughtful revelations. This book will serve as a guide to those who wish to pursue similar goals and undertake similar programs.

The specific union structure, the New York Joint Board, Amalgamated Clothing Workers of America, and the lofts and shops that characterize this industry are not common work settings across the country. However, the contributions of this study should not be underestimated. It will help to dispel two commonly held erroneous beliefs. One belief questions the acceptability of mental care to blue collar workers and the benefits that they can derive from such outpatient services. The second belief is that mentally ill persons cannot work. By restructuring both treatment goals and the work environment, the authors of this book provided the leadership to a mental-health team that demonstrated otherwise.

The authors have skillfully examined their experience. They have distilled and synthesized principles and concepts to offer valuable guidelines for developing mental health services for blue-collar employees. Many aspects of this study can be adapted to other settings, including the community mental health centers which were just beginning as a major force on the American scene when these energetic professionals began their project. During the period of NIMH project support, these authors shared their experiences and findings through a series of articles in journals, papers delivered at professional meetings, and generous consultation to other interested professionals, unions, and business firms. This book consolidates and further illuminates their program and research. It continues to reveal the clarity, perception, sensitivity and high standard of excellence that has characterized their work and their writing.

The National Institute of Mental Health is proud that its Applied Research Grant Program contributed financial support to this important and significant undertaking.

BERTRAM S. BROWN, M.D.
Director, National Institute of Mental Health
United States Department of Health, Education
and Welfare

Preface

This is the story of a journey toward better mental health care for working men and women. In many ways it can be called a dreamer's journey, for among the cast of characters were a group of professionals—social workers, psychiatrists, psychiatric nurses—who dreamed that workers could and should receive better care for their emotional problems.

But it is also a journey of practical men and women, for everyone involved, in varying degrees, recognized the existence of a problem and had some investment in its solution. The events took place in the men's and boys' clothing industry in New York City. The issue of concern was how to bring mental health services to a population which most observers agree is under-cared for, under-treated, and at the same time is an under-utilizer of care. The Sidney Hillman Health Center, an out-patient medical clinic under the auspices of the New York Joint Board of the Amalgamated Clothing Workers of America and the New York Clothing Manufacturers Association, provided a home base for the journey. The Health Center's sponsors also became participants in the program. The workers in the industry and members of their families were the patients, thus completing the cast of characters. The story unfolded over a four-year period from 1964 to 1968.

The first year was spent in resisting pressures, making false starts, holding out for the flexibility necessary to assure the fullest utilization of the new resource by the target population. By the end

15

of the year we determined to focus our activity on the obstacles that
mental illness presented to participation in the world of work. We
viewed the men's and boys' clothing industry as a catchment area—
a community in which people work, functioning much like a geographic neighborhood in which people live. This industry was the
terrain for our journey, a relatively uncharted village with its own
population, institutions, values and recognizable boundaries.

These were years of peak activity and experimentation in community mental health. The thrust of the movement was to bring
mental health care to new population groups. The program detailed
in these pages was part of that general movement. Many people
participated in a collaborative effort involving the union, business
firms, community facilities, and government agencies.

The major financial support for this program came from the
National Institute of Mental Health and the Rehabilitation Services
Administration. The helpful counsel and understanding of the
NIMH staff, especially Mildred Arrill and Dr. Simon Auster, aug-
mented the value of the funds the Institute made available.

This study grew out of a prior demonstration partially financed
by the Rehabilitation Services Administration. That agency has
been supportive in all the endeavors of the authors. Not only their
funds, but also their counsel, especially from Dr. William Usdane,
helped shape the Mental Health-Rehabilitation Program. It was
their support and encouragement which served as the impetus for
the researchers to receive a grant from the Social and Rehabilitation Services which finances our present activity in the world of
work. A regional social welfare research institute known in the
Columbia University community as the Industrial Social Welfare
Center, has been established at the School of Social Work. We are
grateful to the Social and Rehabilitation Services, to Dr. James
Garrett and Region II Commissioner Elmer Smith, and their re-
spective staffs, for permitting us to continue along this exciting
road.

This program would not have been possible without entry to a
population. We deeply appreciate the cooperation of Co-managers
Louis Hollander and Vincent Lacapria, New York Joint Board,
Amalgamated Clothing Workers of America, who provided access

to their membership and encouraged the participation of their staff. We enjoyed the opportunity of working with the trade managers, business agents, and shop stewards, while benefiting from their guidance. The Director of the Sidney Hillman Health Center, the late Dr. Morris Brand, a champion of new rehabilitation services for working Americans, contributed immeasurable support to this venture. The staff at the Center provided back-up for our activities as well as a warm welcome for us. To all these dedicated men and women, we express our thanks.

The data bank which the Amalgamated Insurance Fund made available to us proved an excellent source of baseline demographic and income information. For that, and the constant cooperation available from the Fund, we thank James Shoaff and Dena Wechter.

Emanuel Weinstein, President of the New York Manufacturers Association, and numerous individual manufacturers extended help to the project and to their individual employees in need, thereby influencing the outcome of the program.

Links with selected community facilities were vital to the success of this project. The relationships developed with Mt. Sinai, St. Vincent's and Maimonides Hospitals, and the back-up services they offered, made innovation possible and permitted experiments with different divisions of labor. A special contribution was made by Dr. Burton Nackenson, who functioned as the on-site liaison psychiatrist from Mt. Sinai Hospital.

The early formulation of the idea for this program was influenced by the advice of Bertram Black and Terence Carroll. Continued valuable help and insights were offered by the Advisory Board of this program, comprised of Doctors Iago Galdston, Alfred Kahn, Louis Linn and Leo Srole and Mr. Allen Williams.

The spirit which made this demonstration a vital and inspiriting one resulted from the élan, dedication and competence of the core staff which, in addition to ourselves, included the Medical Director, Dr. Robert Navarre, whose approach to psychiatry helped shape the general thrust of this program, and Antonio Blanco, Edna Coleman, Anne d'Este, Ruth Esterowitz, Rose Lewis, Yetta Ostrow, Dr. Elda Patton, Dr. Jaime Titievsky, and Nilsa Velez. In addition, students and other staff members participated in the program during various periods of operation, and we express our gratitude to all of them. To Yetta Ostrow we offer particular thanks for the care with which this manuscript was assembled and typed.

Although the exciting program which unfolded in the men's clothing industry was the product of collective effort, the authors bear sole responsibility for the interpretation presented in this manuscript.

HYMAN J. WEINER
SHEILA H. AKABAS
JOHN J. SOMMER

MENTAL HEALTH CARE IN THE WORLD OF WORK

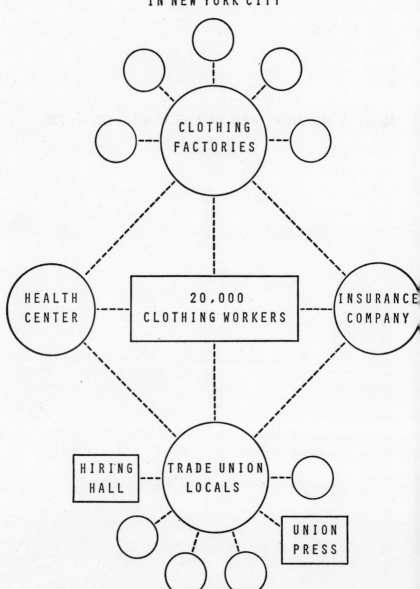

FIG. 1
MEN'S AND BOYS' CLOTHING INDUSTRY
IN NEW YORK CITY

CLOTHING FACTORIES

HEALTH CENTER

20,000 CLOTHING WORKERS

INSURANCE COMPANY

HIRING HALL

TRADE UNION LOCALS

UNION PRESS

The Beginnings

The first year in any program is a critical period. Beginnings generate their own dynamics, often determining the course of subsequent events. The notion of "fail safe"—a point of no return—is relevant. The moment arrives after which it is impossible to extricate a program from that which is already committed, carried out, done.

This program was framed as a new approach to delivery of mental health care for blue-collar workers. Our plan was to involve the entire community in an industry-wide approach to locating and servicing the needs of the mentally ill. Yet for all our understanding of the importance of involving the industrial auspice, the experience of the first year was a history of being pulled toward the traditional way of finding people with emotional problems. We emerged from the first year with a much more sympathetic understanding of the reasons mental health programs in a variety of settings and under heterogeneous circumstances often tend to develop case-finding channels which look alike.

Initial Problems

Objectively, the new clinic faces a field in which certain long-standing pulls exert their inevitable attraction. There are always people in trouble who need care. At the beginning of our own program we were faced with a backlog of potential patients with emotional illness. Eighty-eight such cases of union members, their wives or children were brought to the attention of the clinic in the first two months—almost before staff was recruited and surely before program direction was developed. Such an early caseload, many with chronic problems, brings a demand for service which quickly erodes available time. In short order, patient and professional tend to get locked into a symbiotic relationship which threatens the availability of time for developing new ways of reaching people and serving the functional community of their world of work.

The demands of long-ill patients were paralleled in our experience by another, equally powerful dynamic. Our commitment to innovate by creating new relationships between representatives of the world of work and the mental health clinic was equally threatened by the apprehension of the industrial partners—labor and management—about becoming involved in a hitherto taboo area. Though professionals like to cast mental illness as just one more medical problem, in reality mental illness is not like any other illness. It calls out fear, suspicion and denial which result in institutional resistances. This, in turn, can lead to potential isolation of the mental health clinic from the industry and its constituents.

Nor was this response completely unfounded. For example, during the time of planning and waiting prior to the receipt of the grant for the mental health program, the union leadership expressed considerable concern about how their own reference group would view such a grant. Needless to say their worst fears were confirmed. Announcement of the award was followed by congratulatory, tongue-in-cheek calls to the Joint Board leadership from their co-unionists. As reported to us, the tone of these calls went something like this: "Congratulations. It's a good thing you got the money. I always knew your tailors were nuts!" Can the industry's leadership be blamed for being worried that, beneath the humor, lay a grain of truth?

Good will and working relationships between professionals and labor and management representatives had been built up during an earlier program concerned with rehabilitation of the physically disabled.[1] While the good will remained, it became clear that the

_____

1. See Hyman J. Weiner, Shelley H. Akabas and Bruce Grynbaum, *Demand for Rehabilitation in a Labor Union Population: Part One: Research*

working relationship would not withstand, unscathed, the transition to helping the emotionally ill. The basis for collaboration had to be renegotiated around the issue of mental health. Otherwise, the clinic would find itself in a satellite position isolated—as clinics so often are—from its functional community, the men's and boys' clothing industry.

The pull toward providing services only for those who reach the program through traditional channels is further exacerbated by the fact that our program derived from a time-limited demonstration grant. There developed a sense of urgency to produce within the allotted time. A drift toward action rather than deliberation and planning resulted. Provision of immediate clinical care threatened to shift the primary program focus from testing out new delivery systems.

Fortunately, the program did not ultimately succumb to these powerful influences. The research requirement of the grant helped focus our attention on a search for critical areas in which we might contribute knowledge to the field of mental health care. In casting about for such a dimension which would, at the same time, run congruent to program development, we set in motion forces encouraging to the development of definitions and approaches appropriate to the industrial terrain. The early months were also spent constructing a monitoring and evaluation system with two important dimensions; creating communication within the work group and developing an ongoing information gathering and feedback mechanism. During the prior three years the core staff had struggled to arrive at a style of open discussion. They were able to raise disquieting questions about each other's work. Collective problem solving minimized the feeling of personal attack in such confrontations. New staff members became socialized into this interaction pattern. The resulting climate permitted the group to make appropriate use of the monitoring system's indications that the program was off course despite the threatening nature of such information.

Report (Sidney Hillman Health Center, New York, 1964) and Hyman J. Weiner, *et al., Demand For Rehabilitation in a Labor Union Population: Part Two: Action Program* (Sidney Hillman Health Center, New York, 1966).

This atmosphere helped establish the necessary preconditions for the project to develop its "own thing." Almost from the beginning, a central question guided the deliberations, namely, why should a mental health program exist in an industrial setting? [2] It was by constantly focusing on this question that we were led to a definition of our *raison d'être*.

The World of Work as a Community

The uniqueness of an industrial setting is that its community membership is made up of workers, its community goal is production, its community power resides with institutional representatives of management and labor, its community culture reflects the ethnic backgrounds of its constituents.

An industry-based mental health program, to justify its existence, must reflect, in both form and content, this unique character of its work environment. Operationally, this meant that we viewed the men's and boys' clothing industry as a functional community. The program had to be relevant to the industry. The power forces had to be enlisted to legitimate the goal of the program.

This in turn forced us to focus on the goals a mental health clinic could properly have which would be sufficiently relevant to gain sanction from the industry's labor and management. A strategy was evolved which would tie the clinic to its institutional world. Primary service was offered to those clinic entrants who, as workers, found that their emotional illness was in some way presenting obstacles to satisfactory performance on the job.[3] Our goal for these patients was to maintain them on the job or return them to work whenever possible. This intimately related the clinic to the industry. Collaborative tasks evolved automatically. Instead of mental health care being an activity peripheral to the employment portions of the patient's life, this progam moved the world of work

2. We are grateful to Iago Galdston, M.D., for initially and constantly posing this question for us at the deliberations of the project's Professional Advisory Board.

3. Other applicants for service, especially family members, were offered evaluation services. Thereafter, they were referred to those facilities in the larger community which were more appropriately concerned with the psychiatric problems presented.

"front and center" in the treatment process. Enlisting the representatives of the work community (peers, supervisors, union agents) gave all a stake in the care of each patient and in the success of the clinic in general.

Everything for the next four years flowed from this cardinal decision to cast the clinic as a mental health program concerned primarily with the worker and the obstacles to his continued employment. This rehabilitation philosophy became our North Star, guiding our journey. The selection of this star as our guide represented a successful struggle against several strong and conflicting pressures. We had rejected the ideological pull of those who felt our purpose should be to "decontaminate" the industry so that better mental health care might flourish. The advocates of this view cover the intellectual gamut from those who feel mental health is impossible as long as individuals must perform "alienating jobs," to those who feel that mental health can be achieved in the workplace through certain human relations techniques. We sidestepped the issue of the causal relationship of work to mental illness and concerned ourselves with the more modest goal of helping those whose existing mental illness was an obstacle to maintaining functional performance on the job.

Concern with institutional policy therefore flowed only from our interest in rehabilitating the mentally ill. Individual cases rather than theoretical generalizations were the source for illuminating the existence of problems in the social environment.

The methods and timetable for processing insurance claims, policies regarding job protection and attendance requirements, health center diagnostic and work-up activities were all challenged when institutional practice was found in conflict with patient need. To have any impact on these problems, once identified, required that the mental health program establish a clinical stance as an independent professional operation, representing neither management nor labor.

In an industrial environment, where two power forces are constantly vying for the upper hand, such independence is not easily achieved. Nevertheless, we held firm, refusing to become anyone's agent. We sought the areas of common interest between the industrial partners and the professional team, always with a view to achieving the objective of mental health care for the emotionally ill worker. Out of the struggles to apply these definitions, the clinic described below evolved.

Whom to Service

Experience with patients nudged us, often dramatically, along our path. In fact each case became an opportunity to understand and involve the industry's arrangements and achieve reciprocity between the treatment needs of the individual and the institutional needs of the functional community. The earlier question of "Why should a clinic exist in an industrial setting?" had to be made operational on a case-specific basis. The core question in relation to each referral became, "For whom and in what way is the illness a problem?" Mental illness, per se, was not automatically assumed to be an appropriate problem for this clinic. Only when the answer involved both the patient and his connections to the world of work did the individual meet the criteria for ongoing care by the mental health program. Others were evaluated and referred to outside facilities. Mrs. Jane Clark's [4] situation illustrates the implications in terms of referral and evaluation process and the issues it raises for clinical, administrative and research activity.

Initial project awareness of a possible patient came when Mr. Frank Lovengo, a business agent,[5] mentioned to project personnel a worker whose recent behavior had been moody, causing difficulty in the shop. The business agent, responsible for the shop, regarded Jane Clark's trouble as a potential cause of strain in the factory, making his job more difficult. Shortly thereafter Mr. Lovengo's concern was confirmed by a call from the employer, angrily reporting that Jane, the only ticket sewer in the plant, had stormed out of the shop, upsetting the whole production line. He held Mr. Lovengo responsible, as indeed the union itself does, for cooperative behavior on the part of the organized labor force.

---

4. All names are fictitious while all cases are substantially accurate, modified only as necessary to protect the identity of the patient.

5. A business agent is a paid full-time employee of the union who is assigned the task of handling union-management relations in the group of shops designated for his supervision.

The business agent contacted Mrs. Clark who reported she was angry because "workers were making faces at me." He told Jane her behavior might endanger her job. He recommended that she visit the mental health clinic newly available at the Health Center. In fact, he set up an appointment for her that very evening. She returned to her job the next day but did not keep her clinic appointment. This response alerted the clinic to the fact that the worker's illness was a problem for the union, for the employer, for her co-workers—but not yet for Jane!

The clinic became involved in a consultative role to develop a strategy for ways of involving this worker, who was obviously sick. This outreach activity, to turn an individual apparently needing help into a patient willing to seek help, was possible because of the special way the clinic was related to the institutional world which comprised Jane's work environment. Project personnel advised the business agent that Mrs. Clark had not kept her appointment. They suggested that if she caused or experienced further difficulty, he should not shield Jane from the consequences of her action. Rather he should emphasize the reality—her job was in jeopardy if her disruptive conduct continued.

By the next afternoon, Mr. Lovengo was again called by the boss because Mrs. Clark threw a piece of metal at one of her co-workers. When Mr. Lovengo asked Jane about her broken appointment she reportedly said, "If I kept it you would think I was crazy." Mr. Lovengo replied, "I don't think you are crazy. But I know you are going to lose your job." He later reported to the project that he put his arm around her and said, "I'm not talking to you as a brother to a sister [brother and sister are terms used in the union to denote male and female members], but as a father to a daughter —you have problems and you need help now." When Jane still hesitated about coming to the clinic, the business agent offered to accompany her immediately. He called to alert us to the fact that he was on his way with the patient. Although business agents had been confronted with problems like Jane's over a period of years, we found they grasped at the new mental health program as a more viable alternative than anything previously available for dealing with the disturbed employee.

The case had now passed through a phase which defined "for

whom and in what way is the illness a problem?" Originally the employer had defined the illness as a problem to his production process. Her co-workers had defined the illness as a problem to their personal safety. Her business agent had defined the illness as a problem in his relation to both the employer and the workers he represented. Because of these definitions the clinic understood that, potentially, the worker was an appropriate patient for its functional rehabilitation approach.

As the situation unfolded, Jane became aware that from the point of view of her maintenance on the job, her illness was not just a problem for the union, the employer, and those in her workplace, but for herself as well. At this point the clinic was able to move into the case as an independent force. Being the agent of none, it became possible for the mental health program, through a mediating function,[6] to become the agent of all.

The Mediating Function

Mediation assumes an interdependence among the parties which gives each an investment in coming to a collective solution. As a worker Jane is in an interdependent relationship with her employer and as a producer her employer is in an interdependent relationship with Jane. As a worker she is also in an interdependent relationship with the union, the legal representative of Jane at the workplace, and as a membership organization the union is in an interdependent relationship with Jane as its member. Basically, each of these interdependencies stems from Jane's role as a worker. The clinic focused on human beings, not as sufferers but as workers unable to work as a result of an emotional disorder. This places the clinic in a service relationship not only to Jane but to all the interlocking dimensions of Jane's work situation. It affects the definition of the problem for the clinic, both in terms of service

---

6. A model of the mediating technology is set forth in James D. Thompson, *Organization in Action* (New York: McGraw-Hill Book Company, Inc., 1967), *passim,* and in William Schwartz, "The Social Worker in the Group," *The Social Welfare Forum, 1961,* (New York: Columbia University Press, 1961), pp. 146–77.

and research activity. Specifically, three central issues emerge, namely:

—selection of information,

—designation of who is to get involved in treatment,

—choice of what division of labor will accomplish the rehabilitation goal.

In order to service these three dimensions, the clinic needed to be keenly aware of the way of life of the men's and boys' clothing industry. The administrative arrangements of the clinic, therefore, were designed to reflect the charge to the clinic and the nature of the setting and its labor force. They will be detailed in the next chapter.

2

The Clinic Emerges From Its Community

The Industry

The way a program functions is influenced by the environment in which it operates, the product it offers and the technology it utilizes. The goal of this clinic—its product—was to provide mental health services to emotionally ill workers to help them maintain themselves on, or return to, the job. We adopted a mediating technology of bringing together the parties to identify and deal with the obstacles to continued employment. The setting of the men's and boys' clothing industry, with its production function and institutional network, constituted the program's environment.

The clinic reflected the style of life and rhythm of the industry. For most representatives of this world, union or management, time is money. Every personal act and environmental occurrence has a price—the more demanding the act or time-consuming the incident the higher the cost of being involved. When Jane Clark threw something at a co-worker, she represented a cost which could be minimized only by speedy action. Other industries might be able to tolerate a sedate response to illness. But the highly competitive piecework atmosphere of men's clothing manufacturing means that a clinic with the usual intake procedure and waiting list would constitute too costly a solution pattern. By the time the contact would have been established with the typical mental health service the garment manufacturer would have secured another ticket sewer and neither management nor labor would be interested, any longer, in investing valuable time in helping Jane.

We interpreted our mandate to service the mental health needs of Jane and her co-workers as a charge to establish a treatment facility consistent with the demands of her industrial community. A crisis-oriented rehabilitation clinic enabled staff to move quickly toward the goal of maintaining someone at work. It also was consistent with our philosophy of service to maximize the involvement of significant others in the treatment process.

This industry, the functional community in which our potential patients worked, has, like any community, a unique and long-established culture and social structure. The manufacture of clothing was one of the first industrialized areas in society. Its technology has not changed very much since it began. It depends on a labor force which contributes manual skill to the production process. The average worker sits at a sewing machine putting together a small section of a total garment. The more sections he puts together, the higher his earnings since he is most likely to be working on a piece-rate system of payment. His workplace is usually an old loft where anywhere from one to five hundred of his co-unionists labor. There is a great diversity in shop size—a majority of the firms have fewer than ten workers, but a majority of the workers hold jobs with employers of 100 or more. Altogether about 20,000—47.6 per cent men and 52.4 per cent women [1] labor to manufacture a portion of the suits and coats and outerwear that men buy each year.

The Workers

All the workers are members of the New York Joint Board, Amalgamated Clothing Workers of America. The majority (60 per cent) represent the early Jewish and Italian immigration which flooded the industry in the first years of this century. Although the Jewish population has diminished yearly and is now about 15

---

1. These and subsequent figures on labor force characteristics are estimates developed from intensive study of a 5 per cent random sample of the workers employed in March 1967.

per cent, the Italians who have continued to enter the industry make up some 45 per cent of the labor force. The remaining 40 per cent includes representatives of such heterogeneous ethnic groups as Puerto Ricans, American blacks, Greeks, etc. In fact, in this industry ethnic is everything, or almost everything. Shops, from owner on down, are often organized along ethnic lines and the union leadership reflects this ethnicity. The ethnic composition of the industry has a profound impact on all arrangements therein from who gets what job to the economic and social supportive systems, not the least of which is the degree of tolerance of deviance at the workplace.

The workers in this industry are a little different than the prototype American worker. The vast majority were born outside the continental United States (72 per cent) and in part, as a result of this foreign origin, tend to be less educated than the average worker. The median education completed by the garment worker is grade school, while for the economy as a whole the educational attainment of the median worker is high-school graduation. For many, employment in this industry is regarded by them as the best of available alternatives. Not surprisingly, therefore, the workers exhibit a high level of attachment to their jobs and the industry.

Eighty per cent have worked in the industry more than five years; and 63 per cent of this group have been with the same employer for at least that length of time. This long-term tenure is, in part, a function of the age distribution in the industry. The median grouping is in the forty-five to fifty-four age range, one decade older than the national figure. Since according to labor force studies age is highly correlated with job stability, this tendency to job attachment can be explained, at least in part, on the basis of an aging labor force.

The essential statistics outlined above provide a cross-section view of the industry's work force at a particular point in time. The trends over time, however, are important for an appreciation of the atmosphere in which the mental health program developed. In fact, we found ourselves operating in a period of rapid industrial transition. Small shops were giving way to the national movement toward consolidation. Ethnic majorities were being eroded by new labor force entrants. The basis of the empathy resulting from employers of the same ethnic group as the workers, from union leaders of the same sex and ethnic group as their members, was diminishing. There was an onslaught of women, outnumbering the former male majority, and a radical redistribution of the ethnic composition of the labor force. The Jews, earlier the dominant cluster, became a vanishing breed of workers, yet still held an aged hand on the reigns of union leadership. Italian workers were moving to the fore as they continued to replace their retiring numbers with young immigrants and middle-aged women. The remaining openings in the industry were being filled by still other foreign-born, primarily Spanish-speaking, young females.[2]

"Bread and Roses"

The historical tendency in the industry had been for the union to be the central force. It was the union which had brought productive order out of the chaotic conditions resulting from competition among many small producers. It was the union which had customarily recruited the labor force for the industry from among its ethnic constituency. The increasing scale of manufacturing operations and the changing ethnic nature of the labor force has tended to dilute, somewhat, the position of the union. It continues to exercise significant power within the industry because of the union shop provision in the contract. Nationally its ongoing leadership as a labor organization dedicated to the concept of social unionism assures it a respected position in the AFL-CIO. The goal enunciated for the Amalgamated by its first president and distinguished American leader, Sidney Hillman, was that a union helps its members gain "bread and roses." The Amalgamated continues to enlarge on this heritage as it moves forward in cooperative housing, banking, insurance, day care and health services. Clearly, such a union and the industry which has been its site for over fifty years is potentially hospitable to the creation of a person-oriented service.

In the past, the industry has made some attempts to provide direct services to individuals. The Sidney Hillman Health Center itself represents a joint labor-management endeavor in this direc-

2. Not only Puerto Ricans, but large numbers of immigrants from both Cuba and South America have become garment workers in recent years.

tion. Our own earlier rehabilitation program had provided direct care to the physically disabled. As part of that program we had carried out a specific study of the facilities utilized by the membership. We found a dominant tendency on the part of the population to utilize private physicians. Their use of public agencies was limited, as only 4 per cent of the physically disabled had been in contact with a community facility.[3] What care was utilized was usually illness-directed. Rarely did anyone seek out preventive attention for his physical or emotional problems. It was our impression that much of the behavior and choice of preferred treatment were influenced by group values. The paths to care were often those previously trod by an ethnic peer or co-worker.

One such service, the Sidney Hillman Health Center, provided a significant dimension of the environment in which the mental health clinic operated. Not only did it house the program, but it established the medical model as a framework for our own operation. This model was consistent with the population's preference to regard its problems as medical rather than personal and with our definition of presenting problems as crisis situations rather than chronic conditions. On the other hand, the center's rigid hierarchy introduced strains for nonmedical personnel which interfered with the mental health clinic's search for egalitarian professional status among the psychiatrists, social workers, psychologists, nurses and administrative personnel who comprised our staff.

Clinical Arrangements

As we embarked on the development of the mental health program, we attempted to capitalize on this knowledge and understanding. An administrative structure was evolved which was designed to reflect the needs of the industry, its belief systems, and the help-seeking patterns of its labor force. Original procedures were further refined in the process of providing direct service to patients with emotional illness. What finally took shape was a clinic which offered optimum accessibility to the patient and the

---

3. Hyman J. Weiner, Shelley H. Akabas and Bruce Grynbaum, *Demand for Rehabilitation in a Labor Union Population: Part One: Research Report* (Sidney Hillman Health Center, New York, 1964).

significant others from his world of work. We started by recruiting multilingual staff members and then making them available at times convenient to the patient and his work schedule. Therapeutic personnel saw clinic clients on lunch hours, in the evenings and before work started in the morning. Of the 442 patients eventually seen by the clinic many came to our door unannounced and found a professional ready to talk with them, if only for a few minutes. More sustained contacts were arranged for very shortly thereafter. Nor was the office considered sacrosanct. Staff members were available to see patients at their machines, in local coffee shops, at the union hall or any place else to which they were called. Often these calls came from institutional representatives of labor or management to the specific staff member who had been assigned to service that arm of the industrial network. Administratively, a division of labor was established within the program's professional staff to guarantee to the various industrial arms the same easy access which we provided to the patients. One staffer became expert at insurance problems, another worked in liaison with the union's hiring hall, a third developed a special relationship with the segment of the industry involved in shirtmaking, etc. The arrangements helped to establish the kind of relationship which maximized trust—trust between the program and the institution, between the program and the patient, and between the institution and the patient.

These easy access provisions were, in essence, designed to minimize stigma for the individual who was seeking or needed help from the program. Another set of administrative arrangements was geared toward maintaining the individual in treatment and helping him remain at, or return to, gainful employment. These fall into four overlapping areas, and were designed to maximize the use of available resources in light of the work goal, namely: (1) coordination of treatment effort, (2) collection and use of information, (3) rhythm of treatment, and (4) program accountability.

For the new patient, a professional was assigned to function not exclusively as a therapist but also as a coordinator to see that the individual received all the clinic could offer. This coordinator enlisted as many actors as necessary to assure that those who should be engaged in helping the patient were so engaged. Selectively, he involved the patient, his family members, his business agent, employer, co-workers and other mental health clinic staff members. When necessary, the coordinator could make use of services at three hospitals [4] with which the clinic had established contractual relations and with other facilities in the community at large. Thus, the team was flexible, often open-ended, included indigenous industrial personnel, and provided opportunity for clinicians other than the patient's coordinator to participate when indicated. The patient, on his part, came to view many on the staff as his personal helpers.

Our primary purpose was always to help the patient make an adjustment to his work world. Information became a vital ingredient in this effort. Securing information was framed immediately as a collective task. A person's problem, as it affects his job, is not a secret. Everybody in the factory knows about it. The mental health clinic helped maintain this climate of openness by moving quickly and matter-of-factly in terms of gathering information. Therapist, patient, labor and management representatives each contributed what he could. Whether the information was subjective or objective was irrelevant. It was the coordinator's role to put together a picture of the patient, his perceived and real problems, in relationships with his peers and supervisors, his ability to perform occupational tasks and to meet the demands of his work routine. Relationship, task performance and ability to adhere to routine became the pivots upon which to evaluate the mental health problem faced by the new clinic entrant.[5]

Administratively, we adopted an intake interview instrument which was developed jointly by research and clinical personnel. It provided for systematic recording of specific information on the patient vis-à-vis his world of work. This focus was intended to keep the therapist-interviewer from straying too far afield into intra-psychic matters unrelated to the presenting problem. It also assured parallel information on all patients for later research analysis.

---

4. The cooperating hospitals were Maimonides Medical Center, Mt. Sinai Medical Center and St. Vincent's Hospital in New York City.

5. See Walter S. Neff, *Work and Human Behavior* (New York: Atherton Press, 1968), for a discussion of the interaction among routine, task performance and interpersonal relationship in relation to work.

Embodied in the instrument was a release form which patients were asked to sign so that we might continuously gather information from all relevant sources throughout the service period of the case. The data became the basis for an ongoing feedback mechanism which improved communication among the team participants and permitted joint and relatively speedy problem solving based on reality information. (See Appendix A for the Intake Interview Form.)

The dynamic nature of the information retrieval process was just one ingredient of a clinic which serviced its patients at a rate of speed comparable to the pace at which suits are produced. We started from a premise that every patient's treatment schedule should be custom tailored to his own presenting problem. Both the hours and frequency of treatment were flexible. Face-to-face interviews were interlaced with an open line of telephone contact with significant others in the patients' lives. For all patients the telephone was a significant source of readily available help.

The treatment style varied. One patient saw a psychiatrist and a social worker, another was placed on a drug regime, a third saw the coordinator in the company of his business agent. One patient might come in daily for two weeks and not be seen again until a year later when another problem precipitated a flurry of activity. Another worker might need an evening session weekly for a month or so. Still others were seen only once and carried on alone thereafter with periodic telephone calls to the office. The crisis orientation, rehabilitation goal, and flexible treatment schedule made it possible to service a relatively large number of patients.

Accountability

The reader should not think that the arrangements detailed above were developed at the outset and ran smoothly throughout. The program experienced many crises which threatened its very survival. But the system of accountability which had been built in as a significant dimension of the program helped provide an arena for dealing with controversial issues. In the last analysis, responding to needs is not a simple, clearly defined matter. Rather it is the process of entering into a relationship to develop contractual agreements and guidelines to which all parties can be held accountable.

Participation without accountability is empty, for it leaves undefined the nature of responsibility. Genuine participation requires involvement in the game called "mutual demands."

Although sometimes painful, we sought to establish this game in three sets of relationships, namely: (1) the mental health program with the industry, (2) professional staff with each other, and (3) staff with the patient.

Two mechanisms were created to achieve reciprocity between the mental health program and the industry. First, a policy board representing both labor and management was formed to permit an ongoing dialogue on the relationship of the mental health program to the industry. The board became a place where mental health activities could be sanctioned and resources allocated. The approval of the gatekeepers was critical if firing line professionals were to be permitted entry into the factories, union halls, even local cafeterias, for there were times when their activities infringed on the normal production process. At the same time, the board meetings became the arena for industrial representatives and professionals to raise pointed questions about each other's activities. Why were patients referred to outside facilities? How much information did a manufacturer need for safe employment of a worker on a therapeutic drug regime? Why did a service program need research information? Was government subsidization of employers appropriate for on-the-job training placements? These were but a few of the issues grappled with at these policy sessions.

On another level, a mechanism for case-specific accountability was instituted through a regular interchange between project personnel and the source of referral or other parties significantly involved with the patient. Communication channels were opened with insurance company representatives, managers and foremen, Health Center personnel, and with union business agents and shop stewards. These, most often, were specifically structured encounters where different representatives met on a scheduled basis to operationalize the accountability concept.

On a more individual basis, Jane's case, referred to earlier, provides an example of these mutual demands. When she did not show up at the clinic we urged the business agent to keep close to her and try to bring her in for an appointment despite his own feeling of discomfort in talking to her about her emotional problem. On his part, he required that we be immediately ready to see the patient when he arrived with her at the clinic door despite any dislocation this might cause in work schedules.

The second area of mutual demands was represented in the staff's relation with each other. These mechanisms can best be described as "quality control" procedures. Considerable visibility of each other's work existed because several professionals often serviced different aspects of a single patient's therapeutic program. By the end of the third year, even intake interviews became joint enterprises. Constantly shifting mixed teams of psychiatrists and social workers participated in the first encounter with a patient. At this and other points in the patient-staff relationship, clinicians were charged with the gathering of research information. The requirements established by the research arm served as an additional internal check on staff activity. Finally, collective examination of a patient's condition took place on a regular basis. This guaranteed attention to specific work goals and precluded a therapist's developing a long-term "private case load." Superimposed on this entire framework, however, was the reality that, as a mental health clinic operating in New York State, ultimate legal responsibility for patient care resided in the psychiatrist.

One of the distinguishing features of this clinic was our determination to minimize the magic in the therapeutic process by sharing information with the patient and allowing him into the sacrosanct domain of decision making. This meant that he was often a participant in team conferences. This participation required that goals be mutually arrived at. Patient and staff could hold each other to a plan of action which evolved from their collaboration.[6]

In this chapter we have attempted to portray the flavor of our clinic as it responded to and was affected by the environment in which it operated and the product it hoped to offer its constituents in the functional community of the men's and boys' clothing industry in New York City. The next few chapters will describe the nitty-gritty of the program's operation.

---

6. For a discussion of accountability to the consumer, see the pioneering work in this field, Bertha Reynolds, *Social Work and Social Living,* (New York: Citadel Press, 1951).

Many Paths to Care

A Strategy

Every clinic develops a strategy to locate those for whom it has been designed. Among the tailors of New York, we assumed there were many who just about manage to survive each day, so pressing are the work difficulties they experience as a result of emotional problems. Our clinic sought to reach and service these working men and women whose illness was a problem both to themselves and to the industry in which they were employed. Our strategy was to devise an approach by which the limitations imposed by illness could be minimized and the work role maintained to the benefit of the patient and the institutional parties.

Locating such individuals was, however, not an easy undertaking. Labor and management had to view the mental health service as relevant to their own organizational interests if they were to be involved in the process of finding cases. Workers, contrary to usual blue-collar behavior,[1] had to see psychotherapeutic help as a desirable way of dealing with emotional illness if they were to become patients. Specifically, we proceeded in two major directions. First, we located those points in the institutional arrangement, namely,

---

1. See, for example, August B. Hollingshead and Frederick C. Redlich, *Social Class and Mental Illness: A Community Study* (New York: John Wiley & Sons, Inc., 1958), and I. Zola, "Illness Behavior of the Working Class" in Arthur Shostak and William Gomberg, eds., *Blue-Collar World: Studies of the American Worker* (Englewood Cliffs, New Jersey: Prentice-Hall, Inc., 1964), pp. 351–61.

the Health Center, the insurance company, the union's network and the shops themselves, where emotionally ill workers might be more readily identified, either because those with emotional problems might show up there (e.g. the Health Center) or because those with emotional problems tend to call attention to themselves there (e.g. the factory). We established mechanisms which would help to channel those workers into the mental health program. Second, we sought to legitimate help-seeking behavior. We encouraged the union through its leadership and constituent groups to sanction the pursuit of psychiatric treatment. The essence of our strategy, thus, was to approach and engage the functional community. We chose this route in preference to a program which would attempt, through formal education, to change long-standing help-seeking patterns.[2]

Case finding is the first task in a process of mental health care. It therefore became the first line of our work with the functional community. The way a case originates tends to frame its future course. The typical procedure where the community serves only as the case-finding mechanism and the clinic operates as the exclusive case-treating mechanism was rejected. We framed the helping process as a pooled enterprise throughout, with collaboration beginning around case finding. We adopted a position which defined locating people in trouble as a clinical activity requiring the same investment of professional time and skill as any other aspect of treatment. Particularly for blue-collar workers, identified as often reluctant to seek psychotherapeutic services, the possibility of using the case-finding incident as a concrete opportunity for patient engagement is most significant. Locating the client, then, becomes part of the continuous process of patient-clinic relationship running from origination, through engagement and treatment, to discharge. Further, the interlocking nature of case and community is fostered by this approach. Each worker-patient becomes an expression of the problems facing the functional community and its constituent members, and an opportunity to deal with these problems.

The building of a relationship to the functional community was

---

2. Charles Kadushin, *Why People Go to Psychiatrists* (New York: Atherton Press, 1969).

a multilevel operation reflecting the varied nature both of the case-finding sources and of the cases found. For some workers the mere announcement of the mental health program was sufficient to bring a patient to the clinic, as exemplified by the first wave of chronically ill individuals discussed earlier. For others, some encouragement in the way of personal contact by a business agent, insurance representative or physician was necessary to activate the latent interest in seeking help. The most extensive collaborative effort was required for those like Jane, who resisted recognizing the jeopardy in which their illness placed their economic role. The story of specific referral experience from the various sources will be used to shed light on this complex process of locating and engaging patients. But first, let us pause to provide some boundaries for our discussion.

Social Bookkeeping

In 1964 when this program started much of the literature on mental illness decried the inadequate record keeping in the field. This was identified as contributing to the number of individuals who seemed to fall through the cracks of community mental health services. In response to this, we determined to establish a central registry which would become a confidential repository of the names of all workers and family members who were "reported as having a mental health problem." These reports came from professionals, indigenous nonprofessionals and patients and their relatives. Although it could never be regarded as an epidemiological count of mental illness in the men's and boys' clothing industry, the central registry did provide a gross net to catch people whose problems were seen by themselves or others as deriving from emotional illness. Such a registry also provided an indication of which sections of the industry were reaching out for help and the kind of service demanded. The information required in the registration process supplied a profile of who the registrants were—their age, sex, ethnic group membership, local affiliation, utilization of Health Center and other demographic data. Through it we could pinpoint whom we were reaching and which segments of the population we might be missing. This established a basis for planning our own movements and the allocation of institutional resources. If not enough Italians appeared on the registry, we could visit an Italian local. If too many aged appeared we could let up in our efforts with the Health Center. The central registry thus became a control instrument. It also provided a measure of the impact of our efforts. Finally, it acted as a clearinghouse through which we could check new names and new referrals.

Table 1 below shows the pool of 718 individuals reported to central registry from September 1, 1964, to October 31, 1967, by the source of the referral. It is important to note that only 61.6 per cent of those on the central registry ended up as consumers of service. For 15.7 per cent efforts to pursue them were unsuccessful. Finally, 22.7 per cent were "registered only," and no contact was ever attempted for a variety of reasons that will be discussed later in this chapter.

TABLE 1

INDIVIDUALS IDENTIFIED AS HAVING MENTAL HEALTH
PROBLEM BY SOURCE OF REFERRAL

Source	Number	%
Health Center	234	32.6
Insurance Company	226	31.5
Union	103	14.3
Self or Family	89	12.4
All Other	66	9.2
TOTAL	718	100.0

The Union

Anyone attempting to develop a program within the setting of the men's and boys' clothing industry in New York would soon learn of the significant gatekeeping role of the New York Joint Board of the Amalgamated Clothing Workers of America. Little of importance takes place and certainly no changes in direction are possible without the sanction, no matter how passive, of this labor union. By the same token, once their approval is gained many doors open automatically.

We start our discussion of case locating with the union to stress its central role in the collaborative activity of the mental health program. The number of referrals actually tabulated as deriving from the union understate the organization role even in the case-finding procedure.

A labor union is a membership organization. Some segments of public opinion notwithstanding, union leaders remain in power only so long as they tend to their store—i.e., provide service to the membership.[3] Though the union is primarily designed to service problems of wages, hours and working conditions, it is not unusual for members to seek help with social and/or personal problems. In the New York Joint Board, the business agent, while assigned responsibility for economic issues, is often confronted by these other social and personal needs. Prior to our arrival the business agents were, in fact, dealing with emotional problems. One business agent stated:

All of us used to talk at staff meetings that a business agent can't be only a business agent—just somebody to come in and settle a case or a grievance between the employee and the employer. A business agent has to go deeper a little bit and involve himself with the people in his shop—to gain their confidence and to see what's troubling them.[4]

The development of the mental health clinic merely provided them with a new alternative. The trick to case finding with the business agent, then, was to encourage him to report these potential patients. One business agent summarized his reluctance.

When I first came in on this project I was kind of skeptical. How could I tell someone in trouble that he needs help? Suppose I really get a nut who hits me over the head if I tell him to go to a psychiatrist?

3. Joseph Slichter in "The Direction of Unionism 1947–1967: Thrust or Drift?" *Industrial and Labor Relations Review,* Vol. 20, No. 4, July, 1967, pp. 590–91, has noted, "Unions are bodies politic, and leadership is constrained by that obvious but vital fact. It pervades almost all the leader's actions, for it means that he has to be elected and re-elected . . . he must, in short, be an astute politician if he is to rise and survive. . . . True, the leadership is constrained by socioeconomic forces, and this constraint sets limits to the discretionary power of leadership."

4. *Helping Blue-Collar Workers in Trouble* (Sidney Hillman Health Center, New York, 1969), p. 7.

I was concerned. But it worked out all right. It turned out finding people isn't hard at all, because when a business agent goes into a shop, he knows his people and the way they act—the way they talk when they're well. So you know right away when they're not talking the way they usually do.[5]

The participation of the business agent was assured when his needs as an institutional representative of the union could be fulfilled by cooperating with the mental health clinic. These needs, reflecting the union's interests, fall into several areas:

1. The union is in the market for new personal services which will help maintain the loyalty of its membership.

2. The union is under pressure to maintain an experienced labor force for the industry.

3. The union, in its concern for its tradition and community image as a socially responsible pacesetter, seeks to be involved in pioneering social and welfare programs.

It was with an eye to servicing these interests that the union gave the mental health team access to the places where the mentally ill might be identified. We were permitted into the hiring hall, introduced at union meetings, written about in the union press, invited to present our program before the Health Center's board of directors which included representatives of management and labor, and visited the shops in the company of business agents. The union, thus, became an ever-present, if sometimes silent, partner in all case-finding activities—here as the direct referral link, here by alerting a member in need to the clinic's existence, here introducing management to the availability of our services. Thus, although the case itself might be classified as an insurance referral, a health center case, or a self-referral, the union was often the seed behind the case-locating activity.

Nor was the union's sanction, once won, any guarantee of referrals. Case finding was an ever-continuous activity. The flow of patients, from all sources, was a reflection of the pace of our outreach efforts. Daily contact with business agents, regular attendance at union meetings, frequent visits to shops—in essence constant visibility and sustained interaction—were the ingredients

5. *Ibid.*, p. 6.

of a steady referral rate. Figure 2 reflects the flow of referrals to our program from all sources. The reader's attention is called particularly to the increase in direct union referrals from March, 1966. This marks the onset of a unique program developed with the business agents which will be discussed in Chapter 6.

Health Center

The Health Center, the most significant source for the project, accounted for 234 registrants, 32.6 per cent of all those identified as "having a mental health problem." Positioning within the medical arena, which resulted from the placement of the project at the Sidney Hillman Health Center, proved to have more advantages than disadvantages. Being in the Health Center permitted us to be cast as a *medical* program. Many in this population tend to somaticize the expression of their emotional problems. In fact, we adopted the name Rehabilitation-Mental Health Clinic, stressing the former element and thereby increasing the numbers for whom care from this facility was acceptable. There were, however, certain strains due to our location. The Health Center is related to a particular segment of the population—i.e., the older union members with a mixture of chronic complaints. Our availability sometimes encouraged the physicians to refer these patients to psychiatry as a court of last resort.

The Health Center, nevertheless, was a rich source of cases. Despite the difficult problems of integrating our mental health clinic into the general medical facility, therefore, we devoted considerable time to "courting our own house." In all our attempts we sought to supplement physicians and social service staff as they carried out their own roles rather than usurp their function and relationship to the patient. One important aspect of our collaboration was the constant championing of our clinic by the late Dr. Morris Brand, the medical director of the Sidney Hillman Health Center. Although the existence of the mental health program created strains for him both in relation to his own staff and to the leaders of union and management who served as his board of directors, Dr. Brand never lost sight of the positive contribution psychiatric care offered to his overall approach to medical treat-

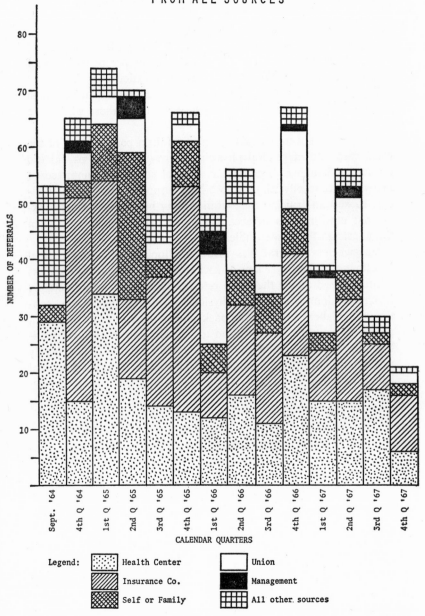

FIG. 2
FLOW OF REFERRALS TO PROJECT
FROM ALL SOURCES

NUMBER OF REFERRALS

CALENDAR QUARTERS

Legend:
- Health Center
- Insurance Co.
- Self or Family
- Union
- Management
- All other sources

ment. His leadership established a hospitable climate for the specific efforts made to approach the center staff, namely:

1. Contact was set up with the social service unit to act as its consultant and treatment source when needed.

2. Working relationships were established with the chiefs of service to help them in their roles as resource personnel for staff doctors who faced complex problems with particular patients.

3. Approaches were made to doctors individually and through a seminar led by one of our staff psychiatrists for those who chose to attend.

These efforts were not always successful; in part because of the usual suspicion of general physicians surrounding any psychiatric service, and in part because the medical staff was comprised of many part-time physicians whose high turnover rate made it difficult to sustain fruitful collaboration. Further, some patients expressed unwillingness to accept a psychiatric referral even when the physician felt it was indicated.

But when a referral was made, it "took"—i.e., the personal investment of the physicians or social workers, as with the business agents, helped assure that once referred the patient would actually reach our door. With those physicians who did participate, continuing collaboration and feedback during the course of treatment permitted simultaneous attention to physical and psychiatric problems—a significant step toward the "total approach" so highly recommended but so difficult to achieve even in community mental health facilities.

Insurance Company

Numerically, the Amalgamated Insurance Company was a prolific source of referrals, accounting for 226 individuals (31.5 per cent of the total) during the life of the project. This nonprofit company is under joint labor-management sponsorship. It functions as the sole carrier for all social insurance provided in the contractual agreement between the Amalgamated Clothing Workers of America and various men's clothing manufacturers' associations throughout the country. Quite unique among bargained programs, mental illness is covered in its hospitalization as well as disability benefits program. An arrangement was established whereby new claims with primary or secondary diagnoses of mental illness would be identified and listed on a referral card and forwarded to the project. This arrangement was possible because the principals of the insurance company and the Health Center were one and the same—the union and the clothing manufacturers. Information, therefore, could be exchanged between them and retain its confidential character. Our procedure was to make at least an offer of service in writing to all persons identified through the insurance company. In 50 cases we actually made attempts to contact the potential patient directly by phone and/or home visit. Claimants were assured that the continuation of their benefits would in no way be affected by their establishing or not establishing contact with the mental health clinic. The fiscal arrangement was thus kept completely independent of the treatment facility. At no time did any patient object to our having been informed of his illness. On the other hand, our reception was not always enthusiastic. It became clear that a machinery geared to dispensing funds was not automatically adapted to transferring trust to a treatment unit.

Eleven per cent of those who became patients of the mental health program had been insurance claimants, but this number is small in proportion to the steady flow of such referrals which totaled over 31 per cent of all those on central registry. The difficulty we experienced in turning these referrals into patients can be attributed to difference in the quality of the cases located through the insurance window. In the first instance, cases lacked the personal link between patient and project of a concerned individual as characterized the union and Health Center referrals. Further, we found that insurance claimants included a heavy proportion of women, many of whom were not primary breadwinners and therefore were under less pressure to return to the employed labor force. Finally, these referrals were identified at a later point in the illness cycle in comparison with the "crisis" referrals which typically originated from other sources. Some had already returned to work by the time they were located, while others were hospitalized and thus under different sources of care.

It is important to note that we had successfully involved a high proportion of the carrier's physically ill claimants in our earlier physical rehabilitation program.[6] In dealing with psychiatric patients our joint case-locating activities never proved as fruitful, despite the excellent cooperation extended by the Amalgamated Insurance Company. Clearly, physically ill claimants have a different perception of offers of service. The ingredient of trust was, we felt, the key to turning Health Center and union referrals into patients. In some way, this ingredient needs to be introduced into the fiscal arrangement if a mental health clinic is to capitalize on this potentially rich source of case finding.

Self-Referrals and Others

In addition to the three major sources of case finding—union, Health Center, and insurance company—a steady stream of individuals made their own way to the clinic, ostensibly self-referred or reported by other family members or patients already under treatment. These cases often reflected the intentioned but indirect influence of the union. The culture of the union which increasingly sanctioned mental health care in its press, at union meetings and in peer group contacts constituted the driving force in a large proportion of the 89 individuals comprising this group. In addition, workers, apparently satisfied with their experience as patients, tended to refer others to the registry.

Of the 66 referrals classified as stemming from all other sources, the impact of the union behind the scenes is again noteworthy. This is especially true of the 33 in this group whom the mental health clinic itself placed on the central registry role. Many were individuals originally in contact with us via the union during the physical rehabilitation program.

Included in this category, as well, were also 16 referrals directly from the industry's management. Just as the union was the silent partner in many referrals classified in Health Center and self-referral, management played a role more significant than the actual numbers reflect. It was often an employer, through his foreman, plant nurse or production manager who initiated the search for care which ended in a union or self-referral at our door.

---

6. See Hyman J. Weiner, *et al., op. cit.,* p. 28.

Though we secured sanction from the official employer organizations, it is fair to say our contact with management was never as extensive as our ties with the union. Each industry has its own distribution of power; its own channels of communication; its own gatekeepers to its resources. In the men's and boys' clothing industry, it became clear to us that the union, based on its control of these factors, was the primary channel for reaching the individual worker. We invested our main resources, therefore, into what we concluded would be the potentially most productive avenue—our relationship to the union.

A long series of historic developments in this industry have brought it to the position where the union asserts and the employers countenance prime control over contact with the individual worker. In another industrial location it may very well be that, although the labor force is unionized, interrelationships do not establish the union as the prime mover.

What is necessary in any setting is to carry out a "social diagnosis." This approach provides insight into the inter- and intra-institutional arrangements which prevail in much the same way as a psychiatric evaluation illuminates inter- and intrapersonal dimensions. The environmental work-up signals the action lines for dealing with the functional community. Case finding, as described here, becomes the first but ever-present grist around which institutional forces can be brought into play. How this is handled determines whether the community-clinic relationship will be collaborative or dependent. Though the specifics may vary, we believe this "social diagnosis" approach can be an avenue for true collaboration and its parallel, division of labor, in many settings—be it a school, hospital or neighborhood. The next chapter will continue our journey from case finding into patient care, along the path established by the collaborative efforts just described.

The Diagnostic Process: A View Through the World of Work

The prime interest of this program was to service those workers who, because of emotional problems, were experiencing difficulty functioning on the job. The availability of the mental health clinic, however, to a population with a variety of needs for care both among themselves and their family members, meant that extensive demands were made on the clinic. Among those seeking service were many individuals who were not the primary targets for service. During the life of the project 718 people were referred to the program. Of these 442 were evaluated and serviced either by the project or a cooperating resource. This chapter will address itself, first to an overview of the patient population and later to a discussion of the rationale and methodology for separating patients into treatment and referral pools.

The Patients

Some characteristics of the clinic population are worthy of note. Table 2, below, shows the breakdown of the patients by diagnosis.

Based on psychiatric diagnosis it is apparent that the clinic population contained a large segment of very sick individuals. Forty-one per cent of the patients were assessed as either psychotic or suffering from organic brain damage. Even the psychoneurotic

TABLE 2

DIAGNOSIS OF ALL PROJECT PATIENTS

	%
Psychotic Disorder	38.4
Psychoneurotic	38.6
Personality Disorder	9.1
Transient Situational Problem	3.3
Organic Brain Damage	2.6
All Other	7.9

population included a larger than usual proportion of acutely suffering individuals.

The substantial numbers of those seeking mental health care for general malaise which appear at many psychiatric facilities did not come to the Sidney Hillman Health Center program. Our patients, rather, sought care at a time of severe crisis in their lives. The rehabilitation philosophy adopted by the clinic grew, therefore, not only out of a research framework, but was actually in keeping with the conditions under which this blue-collar population sought mental health services.

The median age of all patients was in the forty-five to fifty-four age group, a range which included 23.5 per cent of the population. The ten-year groupings, both younger and older, are of approximately equal size marking the clinic population as relatively aged. Of the 442 patients actually serviced, 350 were union members while the remaining were spouses or other immediate relatives. The clinic was never designed as a comprehensive mental health effort. Hence, no claim is made that our efforts reached or identified all or even a cross section of those with emotional problems who were workers in the industry. Nonetheless, it is interesting to examine that portion of the labor force which actually used the clinic. Baseline data is available on the configuration of the industry's labor force along certain demographic and job-related characteristics. It is of interest to compare the union members who used the clinic with the work force in general.

When patients are distributed in the occupational structure, a chi-square test shows them to hold jobs significantly different than those for all workers in the industry at the 5 per cent level but not at the 1 per cent level of significance. Relative to their number in the labor force, patients tended not to come from the least skilled category, but otherwise no clear trend is observable. As noted earlier for the population in general, the sex distribution of the union-member patients is significant. The propensity of males to become patients of the clinic is significant at the 1 per cent level in comparison with the sex distribution of the baseline population.[1] Only 48 per cent of the total of those on the referral rolls were males. Of the recipients of service, however, 58 per cent were men, an unusual statistic for a mental health clinic. The physical location of the clinic in the neighborhood of factory lofts, and its availability during and *after* working hours furthered the sense that it was hospitable to their needs and style. It is our belief, furthermore, that the fact that the union legitimated "going for help" encouraged men, who tended to be closer to the union, to make greater use of the facility than might otherwise be expected. Patients included more young and fewer aged workers than the total labor force in the industry, again significant at the 1 per cent level. Although 12 per cent of the baseline population were over sixty-five, only 3 per cent of the union member-patients were in that age grouping. Nonetheless, there existed a slightly increasing probability of a union member becoming a patient the older he was.

A characteristic which appears to be significantly correlated with patient status at the 1 per cent level is ethnic group membership. In terms of their distribution in the labor force, the Jewish population was more likely to receive treatment than their proportionate position. The Italians were least likely to avail themselves of clinic services, while other ethnic groups contributed approximately their frequency share of the patients. For Jewish workers, the rate of treatment recipients was almost three times their proportion in the labor force, a finding not unlike the experience of other clinics.[2]

---

1. Chi-square is the test of significance used throughout this analysis.

2. See, for example, *The Mental Health Center of the Jamaica Medical Group* (Department of Research and Statistics, H.I.P. of Greater New York, New York, December, 1969), p. 22: "Social status and ethnic group also play important roles as determinants of utilization of psychiatric services. Differences among religious groups are even greater, and the average annual

Not surprising, in view of the ethnic nature of the labor force, is the fact that one patient out of every four required treatment in a foreign language—either Yiddish, Italian or Spanish. The difficulty such patients face in securing "linguistically appropriate" treatment in the community may account for the heavy demand for foreign-speaking therapists at our clinic.

Each characteristic of the patient population detailed suggests its uniqueness—so many men, so many older persons, so many non-English-speaking individuals. In many ways the clinic can be seen as serving those in need who, prior to its establishment, faced only facilities inadequate to meet their need. The functional community of work is, clearly, a significant community through which to reach and service a segment of the society.

Cooperative Endeavors

The clinic was always mindful of its special focus on those with problems which manifested themselves in dysfunctional performance on the job. Yet, it could not ignore the needs of those who sought its services for problems unrelated to the world of work. Links were created with community facilities to augment the ability of the clinic to handle all those requiring care and, most particularly, those with nonwork-connected problems. A variety of patterns were adopted. Sometimes, for example, use was made of hospital insurance benefits to purchase outside services. For the most part, however, these links depended on contractual arrangements with psychiatric facilities at Mt. Sinai, Maimonides and St. Vincent's Hospitals.

While the hospitals were happy to enter into cooperative arrangements, their staff members initially offered resistance to meeting the treatment needs of blue-collar workers. Professionals, intent on the idealized model of a verbal, middle-class patient, often were reluctant to adapt their treatment procedures to a different population. The union, for its part, also offered resistance. Their image of a crowded clinic dispensing "charity care" made them averse to

---

treatment starting rate among Jewish enrollees, 16.0 per 1,000, is double that of Protestant and Catholic enrollees."

having members serviced outside their labor health center. This social distance between institutions in the mental health field and the world of work was an ever-recurring theme. During the course of the program, nonetheless, a number of patients received significant portions of their care from these facilities in a mutual learning experience.

By the end, a represenative of St. Vincent's Hospital was able to comment:

We've been working with the Sidney Hillman Health Center for about two and a half years. I'd like to echo the comment that there's something about the patients who come to us from the Center that makes psychiatric treatment much easier. There's the feeling on the part of the patients that people are interested in them—that they have jobs to go back to—that their concerns are being dealt with on two levels: on the level of the mental health profession, and on the union level.

Essentially, we have run into no problems. We've had our successes; we've had our failures; we've certainly had our experiences. But despite the fact that there's been no screening, no selection by us at all of which patients we'll accept, the patients who've come through the program have, in general, done extremely well.

There's also another angle to the program which is tremendously important to us since we're a training center as well as a hospital. This liaison has helped us acquaint our doctors and our whole professional staff with the labor population and workers' problems.

Psychiatrists have a reputation of remaining pretty much in their office, not being terribly aware of what goes on outside, and I think this has been a justifiable criticism. This program, from our point of view, has been extremely beneficial in terms of breaking down some of our own barriers and misconceptions—we're extremely happy.[3]

And the union, too, had learned that it is possible to work with community facilities.

---

3. *Helping Blue-Collar Workers In Trouble: A Report of a Labor Mental Health Conference* (Sidney Hillman Health Center of New York, 1967), pp. 28–30.

The Evaluation Process

As has been indicated, the clinic saw all who knocked on its door. Clinicians felt that no one should be turned away, but more important, such an easy access policy was in keeping with the style of the world of work and its institutions. Most business personnel offices have an open-door policy. In the men's clothing industry where shops are small, employer and employee frequently of the same ethnic group, and employment relationships long-term, even the "boss" is relatively accessible. Anyone can and does walk into the union hall and, without prior appointment, receives attention. The union "sells" services to its members. A clinic sponsored by such industrial partners could do no less.

The familiar problem of allocation of limited clinic resources, however, had to be confronted. The solution appeared in the form of "switches" on the clinic track. Everyone started out together but after the diagnostic process, those with work-connected mental health problems moved onto the project's "treatment train" while others were referred to community facilities described above. Such referrals were made with caution. The patient was prepared for the referral during as many sessions as were necessary for the project clinician to become satisfied that trust could be transferred. For some, this meant that referral was never undertaken. The key to the referral and treatment process became the diagnostic procedure which separated those with work-connected mental health problems from all others. A few cases may help to describe those who came to the clinic and the differences between service and referral patients.

Tony is a forty-four-year-old Italian employed as a presser for many years. Married, and the father of three children, he has been a high earner in this relatively low-paid industry. In July of 1966, after a minor argument with his foreman, he experienced dizziness, weakness, headaches, sweating and mixed feelings of fear and anger. He became increasingly depressed and decided to stay home because he was ". . . afraid of getting spells—falling on the floor and getting hurt." He began drawing disability benefits from the Amalgamated Insurance Fund, and eventually his name showed up on one of their lists of referrals.

Morris is a sixty-two-year-old former concentration camp victim who for eighteen years had been working as a shipping clerk in a large garment factory. At one point he became so agitated that he struck his foreman. The manufacturer informed the business agent that Morris could not remain on the job. The union's agent took the position that the company could not summarily fire this long-term employee unless he could not perform his usual tasks. The employer and union agreed to have the mental health project evaluate Morris' employability, and jointly referred him to the project.

Juanita is a thirty-four-year-old, Spanish-speaking finisher who had asked her employer for a chance to become a sewing machine operator. The particular unit to which she had requested transfer was composed of Italian workers. Over the months, while she continued to await a transfer, she observed new workers being introduced into that unit and understood this as discrimination against her as a Spanish-speaking person. She began to develop somatic complaints of stomach cramps, nausea and general weakness which reduced her productivity as a finisher. The consequent fall in piece-rate earnings caused her still further anxiety. When she sought medical care at the Sidney Hillman Health Center, the doctor who took the history understood that there was an emotional component to her illness and referred her to the mental health program.

Jim is a forty-five-year-old sewing machine operator who had a reputation for high productivity. A former clinic patient remarked at the change in Jim's behavior on the job when he noticed that periodically Jim would be crying at the machine. For a while he tried to ignore the problem since Jim was able to maintain his production. But when Jim told him about "feeling like he was going out of control" and "an urge to kill a relative, a drug addict who was beating up the family," his co-worker suggested that Jim visit the project.

All these individuals had a mental health problem. Only the first three, however, had a common problem—each was a worker whose psychopathology interfered with his functional role in the work community. *This does not imply any primary causal relationship between work and mental illness.* Often the work environment is relatively neutral becoming only a depository for symptoms. There are, however, also the cases in which the work situation can trigger, exacerbate or magnify pre-existing pathology. Regardless of the starting point, when Tony, Morris and Juanita reached the mental health program they required help in maintaining themselves on the job or returning to work.

When workers are referred to a mental health clinic from the employment situation a new dimension asserts itself. The clinic is concerned not only with the presenting pathology but with *the relationship between the pathology and the individual's ability to work*. The professional staff was quite competent to locate and evaluate the psychopathology. At the outset, however, we could find no clear guidelines to evaluate the interlock of the patient's pathology with his work experience. Contrary to prevailing views we found that there appeared to be no systematic correlation between severity of illness and employability. In fact, we were quite impressed and puzzled by the fact that some patients with major psychopathology were in no danger of job loss, while others with relatively mild presenting symptoms were in serious jeopardy. It became quite clear to the professionals that psychopathology was not the only, or in many cases, the critical dynamic in determining job difficulties. In trying to understand and influence the interface between pathology and functional performance, the professionals found themselves faced with two obstacles: (1) they did not have specific knowledge about the world of work to evaluate job performance; (2) they had no sanctioned power to intervene in the work arena when the course of treatment might so indicate. This reality determined for us that "work as a therapeutic goal" required a new view of roles and diagnostic procedures which was alien to customary professional practice.[4] The interdependence between the clinic and the world of work became apparent. The key diagnostic question became, "What about the symptomatology of the worker, the nature of his work environment and/or their reciprocal impact is precipitating decreasing work effectiveness?" Rehabilitation became a pursuit shared among professional, significant labor-management personnel and the worker-patient. The reader should

---

4. John Sommer, "Work as a Therapeutic Goal: Union-Management Clinical Contributions to a Mental Health Program," *Mental Hygiene,* Vol. 53, No. 2, April, 1969, pp. 263–68.

be aware that the rationale for the clinic stance developed slowly, although it is discussed here in its final form.

Defining the Work Problem

Though there is realization of the importance of "person in situation" information among professionals, the usual diagnostic procedures are such as to leave this issue as secondary material in the evaluation process. The trick was, therefore, to develop an intake procedure which would move to the front of the clinician's consciousness the patient-worker in his work situation and the interplay between the patient and work. An interview instrument was created which served as a watchdog, keeping professionals focused on the employment dimension of the patients. Fortunately, once clinicians began to examine the "patient in work," there were sufficient clinical rewards to continue this consciousness as a style of practice.

The professional's concern during the first encounter is to gather sufficient information to diagnose the patient and identify the first steps in the helping process. The patient, for his part, wants to leave the initial interview feeling better and with a sense that he has come to a place where he will be helped. The objectives of each can be served by concentrating on work information, just as data on early life experience and family relationships contribute vital inputs to the first encounter in other treatment settings. Our patients were blue-collar workers for whom work was an area of relative self-assurance and high interest. By tuning into what was real and comfortable for the patient, the communication gap between middle-class therapist and blue-collar patient could be reduced. The workers we dealt with could see the relevance of talking about work, a subject which was often close to their presenting problem. Historical and family data would have been, for this population, a less acceptable base for establishing contact. The verbal reporting of the patients was encouraged, furthermore, since they were much more accustomed to discuss feelings about work than they were to discuss other aspects of their personal lives. Perhaps most important, an extensive investigation of their relationships and activities at work provided many insights into not only their job performance, but their general functioning.

Always focusing on the presenting problem that the worker brought to the clinic, the intake instrument addressed

—how, if at all, the problem was affecting the patient's work, including the way in which the symptoms were having an impact on job performance;

—what was the patient's history of attachment to the world of work, his present status and his attitudes toward his job;

—who, in the world of work, could be enlisted to provide information and assist with problem resolution;

—what goal, in relation to work, could the clinician and patient address.

The interview form is included in Appendix A. The end product of its use was a functional diagnosis which indicated what the patient could and could not do. The patients' problems were evaluated in behavioral terms and then they were divided into dichotomous groups—those with work-connected mental health problems and all others. Someone with a work-connected problem was defined as a worker,

1) With a positive psychiatric diagnosis based on active symptomatology

2) Affected in at least one of the areas of functional performance of (a) routine and/or (b) task and/or (c) peer and/or supervisory relationships

and either 3 or 4

3) Demonstrated impaired performance defined as

   a) Negative change in production from his own previous work norm

   or b) Perceived self in danger of quitting and so stated

   or c) Had been threatened with firing

   OR

4) Evaluation by team was that prognosis suggested that within 30 days, if untreated, worker would

   a) Experience negative change in his production

   or b) Have to quit

   or c) Be fired.

Conceptually, therefore, we viewed every human being as achieving some type of functional ecological balance. This balance is tenuous for all, but more so in relation to the patient with pathology. Given the individual and his symptomatology, the functional equilibrium of the garment worker is expressed in his skill and task performance, his ability to satisfy demands of the work routine, and the quality of his interpersonal relationship with peers and supervisors. When the balance is upset, be it from a problem outside the work environment or triggered by the employment situation, manifestations of the difficulty appear in these three dimensions of work behavior, task, routine and/or relationship.

Returning to the patients discussed earlier may help elucidate this approach. Tony the presser, suffering from depression, could not meet the *routine* requirement of getting to work. Neither his own work ethic nor his long-standing sense of responsibility as breadwinner had been able to overcome the increasing symptoms of dizziness, headaches, and fear of falling which he experienced. But the interest in having Tony return, expressed by the employer when he was approached for information, became a supportive resource upon which the clinician could draw. This, coupled with the patient's own motivation to accept a goal of return to his job, made it possible for clinician and patient, from the outset, to contract to work toward that objective.

Morris, the shipping clerk with an impulse control problem, was viewed as having difficulty in his *relationship* to those in authority. His suspicious and jealous feelings, inappropriate affect and morbid fears, exacerbated by sharply limited vision in one eye and the constant harassment of a punitive foreman, resulted in his attacking anyone who came at him "in the wrong way." In the face of threatened firings, the business agent, a long-term trusted figure in Morris' life, fought for his job and thus maintained some trust in the patient's increasingly mixed-up world. The agent's commitment that he would be able to marshal a supportive on-the-job network made it possible for the clinician to contract for protection of his job, the dimension of the treatment goal in which the patient was most interested.

Juanita, the finisher who was suffering from numerous somatic complaints, experienced diminished *task* productivity. Her desire for upward mobility on the job was being thwarted, contributing to her sense of despair and anger which she expressed in physical symptoms. The discriminatory aspect of the precipitating situation, once identified, led to an action path. The union's business agent could function as a significant other in resolving the presenting problem by dealing with the discrimination being practiced against her. The goal of promotion, while not eliminating the patient's internal problem, was one she could focus on and which helped to establish trust between her and the clinician.

Jim, whose anger was interfering with his well-being, was in no danger of quitting or being fired. The evaluation procedure revealed that Jim could probably be helped just as adequately at one of the collaborating resources in the community as at the Sidney Hillman Health Center. The goal which he and the clinician set out together was to reduce his feelings of anxiety and impotence. In the absence of a work-connected problem, a referral was made.

Some Dilemmas

The sense of excitement which the foregoing may suggest about the achievements possible for a clinic within the world of work should not mislead the reader into thinking that success was unlimited. The mental health program as a pilot demonstration sought to examine how a clinic could help emotionally ill blue-collar workers maintain employment. This caused clinicians, particularly in the early days, to become trapped into pressing the passive patient back to the work arena before he was ready, or when he was unwilling ever to return.

Besides these individuals who did not find help in the approach outlined, there were difficult issues which arose and were not necessarily resolvable. When the interests of union, management and patient did not merge, the clinic was confronted with the question *"Whose agent is the mental health program?"* This question often expressed itself through the issue of confidentiality and became *"What information needs to be shared by whom to help the patient?"*

The clinic was sponsored by labor and management and, therefore, had to address itself at the very least to some of these parties' sometimes divergent interests. The staff, composed of professionals with a dedication to serving the individual patient, felt constrained, at the same time, to attend to the patients' interests and to act as advocates on their behalf. But being responsive to the interests of organizations simultaneous to the interests of the consumers constitutes a profound professional dilemma. Sometimes a solution is possible by reaching for the common ground between the overlapping needs of organization and consumer, as, for example, when all are interested in maintaining a skilled worker on the job. The clinician serves as mediator, connecting up the interested parties. Such common ground is not always available or possible. When Morris was placed on medication, for instance, the employer sought information on the type of dosage, claiming potential Workmen's Compensation liability as a basis for entitlement to such datum. The clinic adopted the position that only the patient could share such information. In the world of work a further difficulty becomes obvious. Labor and management have an adversary relationship which is sometimes played out in terms of a particular worker. In the case of Morris, the union reacted with rage to management's request for information on medication and there followed a debate between union and management on prerogatives in which the project, unwittingly and unwillingly, found itself in the middle.

Such issues are not easily resolvable. As a guiding principle, the clinic adopted the position of standing with the patient as his advocate and gave up the mediating role when it did not appear to be in the patient's interest. Hopefully, the clinic in the world of work can build up enough trust when it is able to be helpful to all parties so that it can risk acting as advocate when such course is indicated. There were times when it was touch and go as to whether there was enough investment by the parties to assure the continuance of the mental health program in the face of such confrontations.

In the world of work, where one's livelihood is at stake, there is a special significance to maintaining confidentiality since disclosure of information can endanger not only one's personal rights but one's economic survival. Paradoxically, in this setting the usual aspects of the issue of confidentiality loomed less significant than might be expected. The fact that a worker had an emotional problem was an open secret—his employer, work peers and business agent all observed the manifestation of the problem. There was an openness, furthermore, on the part of the patients in discussing their mental disorders. Workers arose at union meetings and announced that they had been helped by the mental health clinic. Patients referred co-workers to the project with the assurance that "they helped me." Letters appeared in the union press thanking the co-managers of the union for providing psychiatric care. These letters would include the signature of the writer. When help was needed from business agent or employer, we would ask the patients if they had any objection to our discussing their problems with labor or management representatives. Almost invariably the union member willingly signed a release to permit us such access.

The issue of confidentiality, therefore, was sometimes turned around to become the clinicians' rather than the patients'. The professional had to establish vigilant guidelines for himself to guard the patients' rights, but not exceed the patients' need for secrecy out of his own professional socialized value system. The balance is tricky, but the clinicians found they could often bend in favor of openness of information without damage to the patient or his rights. Much of this was so because the union, as in the case of Morris, was there to protect the worker-patient's job rights.

This suggests a clinical resource for professionals treating patients outside the work arena as well as within it. Almost one-fourth of the labor force, more in urban areas, are members of trade unions. They *are* the advocate of the workingman and can be enlisted as the advocate of the workingman-patient, especially when employment is threatened in the face of emotional illness.

Though Freud identified the arenas of love and work as the most significant themes of life, only love has received consistent attention from those in the mental health field. The clinic described here was unique in that it was designed to reflect the special needs of those employed in the men's clothing industry. The notion, however, to make work a central focus of the evaluation and, as will be seen later, even the treatment process is, perhaps, an aspect of the mental health program which can be transferable to other clinical arrangements.

Treatment Unfolds:
A Multidimensional Approach

The path to the treatment goal of job maintenance proved multidimensional. It involved gaining experience and accumulating knowledge in four arenas of relatively undefined terrain. It was necessary to ascertain

—how can one locate people in trouble in the world of work who are suffering from emotional problems?

—how does one engage and sustain the involvement of blue-collar workers in the treatment process?

—what is the nature of treatment especially in reference to the unique aspects of psychiatric care vis-à-vis the world of work?

—what should be the division of labor in treatment among patient, clinician, "significant representatives" in the world of work and community agencies?

Answers to these interrelated questions evolved through testing various ways of providing service. The issue of locating cases has been broached in Chapter 3. Here, concern will be with the clinical experience as it began to shed light on the other questions posed. After a review of the nature of the treatment program, several specific aspects of activity will be discussed including the collaborative intake process involving joint interviewing by psychiatrist and social worker, and the use of medication, group therapy and hospitalization.

An Overview of Clinical Activity

Treatment was conceptualized as a process which would help link the worker-patient back to the industrial system of which he had been a part. Face-to-face contact between patient and therapist was the hub around which this clinical activity was organized, but the spokes reached out in many directions. A considerable number of cases involved representatives of labor, management, family and community, separately and in concert. The telephone was a central form of communication, used more frequently in many cases than office visits. Each treatment plan was custom-tailored to the needs of the patient's situation, unique only in that location in industry permitted a wider range of alternatives than is usually available in a treatment setting. The remainder of this chapter will be concerned with the clinical experience of the 350 union member-patients who were treated by the project.[1] Although an additional 92 individuals, all relatives, were serviced by the program, they are not included in this discussion.

Face-to-Face Contact

For a majority of patients treatment was short in duration and involved relatively few face-to-face contacts. Table 3, below, shows the distribution, for each case opening, of the number of individual treatment sessions with professional staff.

The short-term, crisis-oriented nature of treatment is reflected in Table 3. Over three-quarters of the patients were serviced in less than twelve sessions. The remaining required more intensive face-to-face contact with clinicians. Those in the high-frequency tail showed a slight tendency to have a diagnosis of psychotic disorder while those diagnosed as neurotic were somewhat more likely to be in the group receiving fewer direct interviews. The

---

1. These 350 union members accounted for 393 separate case openings in that 37 of them returned to the clinic some time after their cases were closed, 6 of whom had three case openings in total. For statistical purposes, the patient population was handled in a number of ways: sometimes as discrete individuals, $N=350$; sometimes including 2nd openings, $N=387$; sometimes as all openings, $N=393$.

TABLE 3

FACE-TO-FACE INTERVIEWS OF UNION MEMBER-PATIENTS *

Number of Interviews	% of all patients	Cumulative %
1–4	56.2	56.2
5–8	12.2	68.4
9–12	10.3	78.7
13–20	8.5	87.2
21 and over	12.7	99.9

* N= 393

difference, however, is not significant. (For a complete picture of the distribution of treatment sessions by diagnosis, see Appendix Table B-1.)

In essence, the minimal number of sessions is a reflection of the limited nature of the treatment goal—maintenance at or return to work. Clinical strategy was geared not toward a "cure" but toward reducing the symptomatology and/or the environmental stress which interfered with the work endeavor. Given trust and risk taking on the part of the union, management, therapist and patient, an opportunity system results which can incorporate the productive contribution of emotionally ill workers, provided they are free of certain difficulties. The amount of activity, therefore, was not necessarily proportional to the degree of pathology. The issue became, rather, which symptoms, or what in the work situation interfered with the productive role. Clinical care was then proportional to the extent to which symptoms or the work milieu constituted obstacles to employability. There were cases, however, when more intensive therapeutic intervention was necessary even to accomplish the limited goal set out by the project.

Rhythm of Care

As the clinical program unfolded, it was found that patients fell into three basic pools:

1) those who, in a very few sessions, are helped through a

crisis and do not seem to require further treatment to be able to work;

2) those who have a chronic problem but can function well enough except during intermittent points of acute difficulty when they require periodic help;

3) those who required a sustained relationship with the clinic in order to be able to function on the job.

The first category was exemplified by Mrs. Russo, a fifty-three-year-old sewing machine operator who was feeling increasingly isolated and depressed and finally remained home from work. The program reached out to her when her name appeared on a disability insurance list. The sympathetic ear and the medication she found at the clinic prepared her to risk returning to her job. The therapist contacted the shop steward, and together they were able to create, among her co-workers, a receptive climate for her return. She was referred back to a Sidney Hillman Health Center physician for sustained medication after the intervention described was sufficient to overcome the vocational crisis.

Mr. Smith, a thirty-seven-year-old skilled cutter, is more typical of those in category 2, above. He was referred to the project by the union because he believed himself unable to work after a heart attack. Intensive intervention over a six-week period helped him deal with his panic, the level of which was above and beyond what might be realistically precipitated by his physical illness. During treatment, he began to realize that his psychological reaction represented a long-standing response pattern, activated by even minor physical illness. When Mr. Smith felt able to cope with a return to work, his case was closed. A year later he reappeared with similar emotional symptomatology but before employment had been severed. He had learned to identify his need for help and he knew where to turn. After short-term intervention the patient again felt in control of his work situation. Mr. Smith was one of the 37 union members who came back to the clinic more than once in the face of trouble.

Mr. Berman, a chronic paranoid schizophrenic with a past history of hospitalization, was another skilled worker facing job problems. The patient lived in a symbiotic relationship with an elderly mother who, significantly, became ill just prior to Mr. Berman's request for service. He came to the project when auditory hallucinations at work made him sense that he might be unable to continue on the job, an activity he valued as his sole area of independent functioning. He was in treatment for two years and, despite severe mental illness, continued to work throughout. Thirty-three patients, like Mr. Berman, constituted the group requiring long-term treatment even to achieve small gains.

Data on the number of interviews alone does not capture the style of the clinic. An additional dimension of the program's activity was the duration of the relationship between clinic and patient. Two patients with the same number of face-to-face contacts could have entirely different treatment patterns. One, experiencing a crisis, might be seen six times in a few weeks, while another worker with a chronic problem might be seen six times on a once-a-month basis in a supportive relationship. The first patient might be the sole object of clinical activity, while considerable action with industrial representatives might take place in relation to the second.

Unfortunately, no analysis was carried out on length of treatment by frequency of contact. Information is available, however, on the time period during which each patient's case was maintained in service status. This data is recorded in Table 4, below.

TABLE 4

CLINIC POPULATION * BY LENGTH OF TIME IN TREATMENT STATUS

Length of Time	% of all patients	Cumulative %
Less than 1 month	11.4	11.4
1 Month or more but less than 2 mos.	18.3	29.7
2 Months or more but less than 3 mos.	13.7	43.4
3 Months or more but less than 6 mos.	28.9	72.3
6 Months or more but less than 1 yr.	18.3	90.6
1 Year or more	9.4	100.0

* N=393.

Within three months, 43.4 per cent of all patients were serviced and their cases closed. By six months after referral to the program, this total includes almost three-quarters of the clinic's population (72.3 per cent). Sustained contact, nonetheless, was required for a sizable group of all patients (27.7 per cent), including almost 10 per cent who were maintained in a relationship with the clinic for over a year.

It is interesting to note that the skewed tail of long-term patients included, as might be expected, a larger proportion of those with psychotic disorders than those with any other diagnosis. Forty-seven per cent of all workers placed in the psychotic category were in active status for more than six months. For those with neurotic disorders, on the other hand, only 27 per cent are recorded as having a treatment period of more than six months. (More detailed data concerning the relationship between diagnosis and active case status is available in Table B-2, Appendix B.)

The procedures for opening and closing a case are relevant to the reader seeking to evaluate this information. Workers were reported, or reported themselves, to have an emotional problem and be in need of mental health care. These cases were opened when a clinician made a face-to-face contact with such an emotionally ill worker and confirmed his need for service. Such individuals were maintained on treatment status so long as the clinic team judged there to be a role either directly with the patient or with the industrial network. When this need ceased, cases were closed.

Some Clinical Issues

Achieving speedy termination of treatment and acceptance of the limited therapeutic goal based on the rehabilitation philosophy proved to be easier in theory than practice. Clinicians would often develop an investment in the therapeutic relationship which made them unwilling to close the case after dealing with the vocational objective, whether successfully or not. Accountability to a team was instituted. Each month professionals had to justify maintaining a patient in an open status. This built-in control mechanism was not always acceptable to clinicians who felt able to assist patients with problems other than those directly involved with maintenance on the job. Considerable resistance had to be dealt with on a peer level as staff members confronted each other over this issue. Volume of demand, however, more than any artificial criteria assured short duration of treatment. The large number of referrals flowing into the clinic constantly, and the pressure from the industrial parties to have care easily at hand and quickly dispensed, proved to be efficient devices to control duration of treatment.

The vocational rehabilitation approach created still another set of difficulties for the clinicians. Operating in the work milieu sometimes led to an overly enthusiastic response to the needs of the industrial parties, at times to the detriment of the patient's interests. This problem was particularly apparent when a worker was well regarded by the union or management. The case of Vincent Casino is illustrative of this dilemma. Skilled craftsmen were at a premium in the industry, particularly since they were not replacing themselves with younger workers. Vincent was a sixty-seven-year-old expert tailor who was referred by a business agent because he appeared to be upset and unable to work. The agent, in referring the patient, said that he would be extremely grateful if Vincent could be returned to employment because he was desperately needed in the shop.

After several false starts, during which the project assumed that the patient was eager to give up his phobic behavior and return to work, Mr. Casino was finally able to make it clear that he was asking for help in retiring. Because of his long-term relationship with the business agent, and the general ethic of the workplace which defined work as desirable, the patient could not easily indicate that he wanted to retire. Once the patient was able to break through and level with the clinician, helping the project understand his desire for retirement, professional and patient were able to move ahead effectively. The project, however, had to pay the price of helping the worker with his emotional problems. His real need to retire did not satisfy the instrumental interests of the institutions for a skilled labor force.

The debate between those who accept a functional orientation to treatment and those who view improved performance as an outcome of a more extensive treatment plan cannot be resolved by the clinic's experience. All that can be surmised here is that by making clinical activity easily accessible, flexible in hours, short-term, and focused on the work problem, the expectations of the blue-collar consumer merged with the clinical pattern of the Sidney

Hillman Health Center program. The result was that patients seemed to be more easily engaged and maintained in treatment than the literature on mental health care would suggest occurs in the traditional clinic.[2]

The System's Contribution to Treatment

The short-term duration of treatment, with relatively few face-to-face interviews between professional and patient, belies the extent and intensity of clinical activity. The basic approach was to link individuals to their systems and vice versa. The network of resources which was mobilized, and is not available in other settings, was considerable.

The usual cooperation available to a mental health clinic from family members and community resources was, of course, harnessed for the project patients. In 43.2 per cent of all cases relatives were involved in the treatment process. This involvement was in the expected direction in that family participation was enlisted for 56 per cent of all patients with a diagnosis of psychotic disorder and 33 per cent of those patients found to have neurotic problems. The picture is approximately repeated in relation to utilization of community facilities for the project population. A community agency was involved actively in one out of every three cases. For those with psychotic disorders community involvement was achieved in 47 per cent of the total, while the figure drops to 19 per cent among those with a diagnosis of neurotic disorder. (Table B-3, in Appendix B summarizes type of involvement by diagnosis for the union member-patient population.)

The unique ingredient in this program, however, was the use of the industrial network in the treatment process. The union—a resource not customarily utilized to help patients deal with mental illness—was involved in 37.2 per cent of all cases. Here, too the psychotics were the object of a more than proportional share of assistance with the union being mobilized for 44 per cent of all workers diagnosed as psychotic compared with 26 per cent of the neurotic diagnostic category. The most startling figure in this analy-

2. See John E. Mayer and Noel Timms, *The Client Speaks: Working Class Impressions of Casework* (New York: Atherton Press, 1970).

sis, however, is that for 60 per cent of all patients with personality disorders an attempt was made to assist them with and/or through the union. Management, although to a lesser extent, was another unique participant. In 11 per cent of all cases, some employer or his representative was actively involved in serving the patient.

Once a person's emotional problem is visualized in terms of its impact on the functioning of the individual within the environment in which he works, the range of actors in the treatment process is potentially broadened. It extends past the usual dyad of therapist and patient to include all those in the institutional network who are significant to the functioning of the individual or the work community. Industrial representatives possess the knowledge to comprehend the work situation and the power to influence it. There proved to be at least five ways in which representatives of the functional community of work can make significant clinical inputs.

1. *Case finding*—the world of work is able to identify the emotional problem as it is evidenced in deviation from expected performance in terms of task, relationships and routines.

2. *Diagnostic process*—the world of work is able to contribute valuable information about the way in which the emotional problem expresses itself in terms of dysfunctional behavior as well as help identify what in the work environment may "tip the scale."

3. *Referral*—the world of work is able to help in engaging the worker in the treatment process by transferring trust or invoking potential sanctions.

4. *Treatment*—the world of work is able to participate in deciding what environmental modification in the realm of task, routine or relationship is necessary and to seek its implementation including enlisting the support of co-workers. When employment cannot be maintained, the industrial representative also has the power to safeguard a job.

5. *Follow-up*—the world of work is able to serve as the "eyes and ears" of the treatment team directly at the work site.

The Case of Ralph Johnson

The case of Ralph Johnson is an illustration of the multi-faceted contribution of the representatives from the world of work. Mr.

Johnson was a thirty-year-old "kid brother" to six married brothers and sisters. He was still living at home with his mother. He had been out of work for six months. The doctor at the union health center recognized his emotional problems and sent him to the Rehabilitation–Mental Health Program with a request that the clinic help secure a job for Ralph. The patient, at first interview, presented a picture of a character disorder—infantile, self-centered, amoral—and suffering from a sense of rejection by his reference group. He claimed he could not understand why the union and his friends in the men's clothing industry would not help him get his old job back or a new job. He further mistook the therapist's concerned interest as an easy mark for his patterned "con job" behavior. He claimed that the reason he lost his job was that he was too fast—the fastest of any worker. He believed the other workers were jealous of him and somehow this problem of his speed "forced them to get him out." But also evident was his desire to give up the con game because of the fear that too big a price had to be paid. He therefore agreed to have the clinician contact his business agent to find out what the real problem was.

The job reality: The business agent indicated that Mr. Johnson had never learned to be a total mechanic. He could do one or two things very well. He had been working in a very large shop where the work was rationalized and he only needed a small part of the mechanic's skill. It was true Ralph was a fast worker—so fast, in fact, he would make his daily quota by two o'clock and then leave the shop to go to the race track. The union and his fellow workers had informed him that when the boss finally would find out he had departed early (and it was inevitable that he would find out), the employer would rerate the job and make it bad not only for Mr. Johnson but for the other workers as well. The patient had refused to accept this advice, and had openly flaunted the fact that he left early. Finally, the company attempted to rerate the job, and Ralph demanded that the union and fellow workers fight this attempt. When he realized that life could not be the way he wanted it, he quit the job by verbally attacking the union, his fellow workers, and the boss. The union attempted to get him other jobs, which necessitated that he improve his mechanic's skill. He either refused to show up for the job or, when he did, was so incompetent that he was let go within a few days.

The therapist faced the patient with a choice: blame others for his own difficulty and live with the end product of helplessness and fear, or face the reality of learning his skill so that he could be comfortably in control of himself at least at work. Initially, Ralph was angry. He railed at the business agent for misinterpreting the situation; he railed at the therapist for not being on his side. But he finally accepted the message from the therapist that he was free to kid anybody he wanted to, but that he was really in trouble when he kidded himself. Through the union Mr. Johnson took a job where he worked with an old-timer top mechanic who would teach him the trade.

The therapist's statement at the close of the case is of interest.

It is my contention that because the union had a cooperative approach to helping people with emotional problems the following was made possible:

1. The therapist was able to gain quick access to reliable information in a critical area about the patient.

2. The union was able to furnish not only information about the ego (work performance) functioning, but was able to supply the job and training in concert with the therapy program.

3. The union's role of support created the preconditions for the patient, in therapy, to loosen up his defenses of projection and denial and give up some of his infantile behavior.

The Initial Interview—A Shared Activity

An important aspect of a clinic with multiple participants is that patients begin to cathect into not only an individual therapist, but a syndicate of people. In this process some interchangeability of roles develops among the professionals. The clinic decided to promote this aspect of the treatment program by structuring the initial interview as a joint enterprise. The intake instrument discussed in Chapter 4 was administered by a psychiatrist and social worker in concert. This process of a simultaneous interview helped reduce communication problems between the professionals. It also forced both parties to evaluate, together, the interrelationship among the patient's psychodynamics (the traditional bailiwick of the psychiatrist), his social experience (the traditional bailiwick of the social worker) and his work (the traditional arena of neither). After the procedure was in practice for some time, clinicians were asked to comment. One social worker wrote:

I have sensed that most of the patients were surprised and rather grateful for the attention and the length of time they received. This is in very sharp contrast to the rush in medical care that is so common at many other clinics. Many patients were relieved when they learned that one interviewer was an MD and the other a social worker.

Staff's preconceived notion that joint interviews would increase patients' resistance, especially for those with paranoid tendency, was completely ill founded. Following several joint interviews, and comparing them to the individual intake procedure, I began to feel that there was little, if any, correlation between joint interviewing and patient resistance. Essentially the quality of the patient's resistance displays itself the same way whether individually or jointly interviewed. At times I have found that the patient has more of a tendency to let himself go with two people, each playing a different role.

Interesting as it may sound, if there was any resistance it was on the part of the staff and not the patients. In fact, looking back at the time when the idea of joints was introduced, I remember the staff became alarmed. Their immediate reaction had to do with their preoccupation with the effect it would have on the patients. "It will be too frightening for paranoid patients"; "A patient will feel uncomfortable"; "It'll never work with most of the people"; "It could be a waste of time having two people doing an intake." All of this turned out to be staff's projection of their own hangups on joint interviews—a reflection of their own anxieties perhaps related to fear of exposure of one's interviewing style. Some of the clear-cut advantages of the joint interviews are:

1. Saves time.

2. It's less traumatic for the patient to tell the story once instead of repeating it to the MD at a later time during a psychiatric evaluation.

3. Both the social worker and the psychiatrist see the patient in crisis. This facilitates and guarantees immediate planning—case is discussed, recommendations made and plans devised.

4. Plans are discussed and worked out with patient so that the patient doesn't have to wait another week or so or get lost in the shuffle.

5. Immediate diagnosis and planning reflected quick and positive flow which facilitated short-term treatment.[3]

The by-products of having two professionals participate in a single interview, namely, expediting treatment and involving the patient, mitigate the costliness of the procedure. The joint interview permitted a team to get together immediately—consisting of psychiatrist, social worker and patient as the hub and adding individual or community representatives, relatives or Health Center doctors as needed—to direct its attention to collective problem solving. The core team designated the specific treatment dimensions and decided on the need for medication, group therapy and hospitalization—all modalities which were available to the project when needed.

Medication

Medication played a central role in the treatment approach adopted by the clinic. Approximately 40 per cent of all union member-patients received medication as part of their care. For patients, particularly those in therapy with social workers, a psychiatrist was available one evening a week to prescribe drugs and monitor side effects. At the outset of the project, the literature was searched to see if there was any recorded experience concerning whether work, and particularly tasks involved in machine operation, were contraindicated when a patient was on a pharmacological regime, especially in relation to the drugs which staff psychiatrists expected to utilize. There was no evidence of any systematic investigation of this issue, even among psychiatric hospitals with vocational programs. In fact, the only drugs utilized were those approved by the Health Center's formulary committee. That committee, chaired by the medical director of the Sidney Hillman Health Center, adopted a conservative attitude toward inclusion. Only medications with long-standing acceptance in the treatment of mentally ill patients were permitted on the formulary list. Our patients were never experimental subjects in terms of medications.

3. Antonio Blanco, staff member of Sidney Hillman Health Center Mental Health Program, July 25, 1968.

It is noteworthy that employers had considerable anxiety about this aspect of the clinic program, claiming fear that accidents could occur among those on medication. Our psychiatrists maintained that people could work safely at machines while on the drugs which they were prescribing. Under the circumstances, the clinicians adopted the position that prescribed drugs, as any other aspect of the treatment program, were a confidential matter. *To the best of our knowledge, there was not a single industrial accident among the 150 patients being carried on a pharmacological regime.*

The patients, for their part, had mixed responses to prescribed drugs. Many, true to the stereotype of the blue-collar worker, evaluated psychiatric care much like any medical service. Leaving with a prescription in hand made them feel as if they were being properly treated. To our surprise, however, the predominant group held the opposite view—one of deep concern about drug routines. Their reservations included worry that it would become habit forming, that they were giving up control over their own behavior, and that the drugs would produce dangerous side effects. Many saw acceptance of medication as ultimate confirmation of their illness, while some were embarrassed that others might discover they were on medication. Finally, the issue of cost for anyone on a long-term medication regime was a significant problem for this blue-collar, low-income population. *Experience cast doubt on the widely held view that the working man or woman prefers a pill to a verbal exchange.* As with all stereotypes, the grain of truth was not the whole story.

Group Therapy

One of the treatment alternatives introduced midway in the Sidney Hillman Health Center project was a group therapy program. Each group was organized around a common problem, namely, maintaining one's job or returning to work despite an emotional illness. For all other dimensions, great heterogeneity was present among the participants. They were of different diagnostic categories, ages, ethnic backgrounds and sexes, but they were all faced with the common difficulty of "making it on the job." The group constituted itself as a small mutual aid society. Assisted by a psychiatrist and a social worker, they compared problems, helped each other search out new alternatives and adopt modified coping patterns.

Anger is generated in all working situations. Many of the patients, however, had a common way of dealing with their anger; namely, turning it inward. The following excerpt from one of the group sessions illustrates how they went to work on this problem. It began with a statement by Mrs. Valdez:

"Today I wanted to come to the therapy program and my forelady asked me to work overtime. I told her I was going to the doctor. My forelady got me very angry when she said, 'Oh, you're always going to the doctor. Work is more important.'" Mrs. Valdez continued, "I didn't even want to tell her that I go to the doctor. I felt I had to and the forelady wasn't even sympathetic. She was angry at me."

Mr. George then stated, "I understand how she feels. The boss has all the power and he makes us feel like nothing. And I'm sure Mrs. Valdez is frightened of losing her job if she ever said how she feels."

When the therapist asked the rest of the group what they thought, Mr. Frank said, "No, it's not that simple. I think maybe she's a little like me . . . she wants people to like her and she's afraid if she doesn't keep her mouth shut people will get angry at her."

Mr. George interrupted and asked Mrs. Valdez, "Weren't you afraid of getting fired?" Then he asked her what kind of work she was doing. When she identified herself as a sample-maker, Mr. George said, "Oh, that's a very good job requiring a great amount of skill, patience and good judgment. No one would fire a sample-maker, there's such a shortage."

The issue of job loss having been removed, members of the group then came to grips with their inability to handle confrontation both on and off the job. There was an honest sharing of their passivity in the face of anger. Besides sharing information, the session concluded by helping Mrs. Valdez test other ways of responding to the forelady.

It was exciting to observe the culture of the workplace being marshaled for therapeutic purposes. The key contribution of the clinicians was, through focusing on the work problem, to create a climate where emotionally laden material could be honestly shared. The common work environment was the unique ingredient around which the groups were organized. This provided a mutually understandable framework through which individuals could help each other with their problems. Group members met regularly and made demands on each other to alter their traditional responses.

Hospitalization

It was clear from the outset that a certain portion of patients would require a period of time in the protective milieu of a hospital. Fortunately, the health plan available to all workers from the Amalgamated Health Insurance Fund included coverage for 90 days of psychiatric hospitalization. Armed with this fiscal potential, to which the project added a modest grant, the clinic was able to establish working relationships with three in-patient facilities. The primary arrangement was with the Psychiatric Department of Mt. Sinai Hospital, where a contractual agreement was worked out under which one of the department's attending psychiatrists was assigned as liaison to the Rehabilitation–Mental Health Program. He was in attendance at the Sidney Hillman Health Center clinic four hours a week and was also charged with functioning as an ombudsman to expedite hospitalization of patients deemed in need of such care. Of the total of 49 hospitalizations in which the project played an instrumental role, 23, almost half, took place at Mt. Sinai.[4] Gracie Square, a private psychiatric facility, which agreed to accept the Amalgamated Hospital Fund insurance as full payment, cared for seven men's clothing workers, while two others were placed at two other private institutions. A contract, though primarily for out-patient services, was also in force with St. Vincent's Hospital. They made beds available on four occasions for patients. The balance of thirteen hospitalizations were distributed among city and state facilities and the Bernstein Institute of Beth Israel which, at the time, had a new in-patient program for drug addicts.

The recommendation for hospitalization was the responsibility of the psychiatrist. Wherever possible, hospitalization was avoided

---

4. Forty-two discrete individuals were involved in 49 total hospitalizations during the life of the program.

because it meant disruption of work which made the rehabilitation task more difficult. When admission was necessary, however, social work members of the clinic staff often accompanied the patient, with or without family members, to the hospital. Twelve per cent of the 350 union member-patients required periods of hospitalization which varied from a few days to many months. The ninety-day maximum on fiscal benefits often determined the point of discharge, although it was the impression of the projects staff that a number of patients were not necessarily ready for discharge. This "fiscogenic" effect on psychiatric care has been observed by other commentators as well.[5]

By definition all hospitalization cases were work-connected problems. A special "game plan" was activated in their behalf with a view toward achieving the eventual rehabilitation goal of return to work. At the time the case broke, attention was directed at protecting the individual's job rights. This was, perhaps, the most critical feature of the project's involvement since it helped establish the patient's trust and remove a major source of anxiety resulting from hospitalization. It also contributed a basis from which the project could collaborate with the treating institution and served to highlight vocational goals within the treatment plan even of the in-patient facility. Discharge planning, therefore, also reflected the need to lower the person back into the world of work.

Two Illustrative Cases

This dimension of the service program is illustrated by the experience of Mary Balboa. The business agent called the project to refer Mary, who was on the brink of being fired because of excessive crying which began to interfere with her job performance. He described her increasing suspiciousness of co-workers and her expressed feelings that "They're out to get me." On evaluation, it became clear that Mary was in the midst of suicidal thoughts. She responded positively to an offer of hospitalization. The project

---

5. Lisbeth Bamberger, "Financing Mental Health Services and Facilities: Problems, Prospects and Some Policy Proposals," *Till We Have Built Jerusalem* (National Institutes on Rehabilitation and Health Services, Washington, D.C., 1965), pp. 56–81.

called the Mt. Sinai Hospital liaison psychiatrist who determined that a bed was available and alerted the admitting resident to the patient's arrival. At the same time the business agent was called and promised to safeguard her job. This information was shared with Mary by the social worker who accompanied her to Mt. Sinai. Our liaison psychiatrist and project social worker were in constant communication with the Mt. Sinai treatment team. Toward the end of her hospitalization, the project social worker attended a discharge planning conference and agreed to accompany Mary on a visit back to the shop prior to discharge. The business agent was alerted and prepared her co-workers and employer for her return. A week after her shop visit, Mary was discharged, and returned to work. Although she ran into some difficulty, and appeared on the brink of relapse subsequently, the supportive work milieu and the project therapist were able to maintain her on the job.

Early ongoing attention to the vocational issue is a relatively rare dimension in psychiatric care. More usually, social distance and ignorance of each other exists between the representatives of the world of work and those from in-patient psychiatric facilities. It was heartening to discover, however, that given the opportunity, psychiatric staffers were both interested and willing to cooperate with representatives from the world of work. This kind of collaborative arrangement promoted the vocational rehabilitation goal. Smoothing the path back to work, and clarifying and assuring job rights, was certainly helpful to many patients. Having someone who "cares" is especially crucial in helping a hospitalized patient make the transition back to work, as the case of David Warner suggests.

Mr. Warner is a 31-year-old sewing machine operator who has been struggling with impulse control most of his adult life. He referred himself to our program while still regularly employed. After three consecutive weekly sessions with our therapist, he hospitalized himself, although this had not been part of our treatment plan. Following two days' stay in a state hospital, he informed the hospital psychiatrist that he was being treated by us and requested a return to the community under our care. The hospital called; and, in a joint discussion with our psychiatrist, it was agreed that the patient should remain in the hospital for observation and psychiatric treatment.

The patient, however, was concerned about having a job when he left the hospital. He had been unable to inform his employer of his present illness and therefore had not protected his job rights. The hospital could have called the manufacturer, or prepared the patient to handle the call himself. Instead, he signed a release permitting the project to act, and our relationship with the union permitted another alternative. Ongoing contact with the business agent made it possible to share information, frankly, about the patient's problem. The business agent, in turn, called the manufacturer, explaining that the patient's absence was due to a psychiatric illness. The agent indicated that, in the event that the medical situation improved, he would discuss Mr. Warner's return to his job with the manufacturer.

The door to the job remained open because the union was able to assure the patient's job rights.

This simple transaction, when reported to David, strengthened his ego functioning. It demonstrated that he was not alone, that someone cared, that he had a "right" to be ill, that his job rights did not change because of his illness. Further, it removed the burden of his having to protect his own rights at a time when he was too weak to do so. Confirmation by the clinic that security existed in the outside world in the form of a real job reduced the possibilities of secondary gains from continued hospitalization.

At the end of four weeks, the hospital informed the clinic that Mr. Warner was ready to attempt a return to the community. It was felt that this should be tested out while the patient was still officially under the hospital's care. Our staff so informed the business agent who, in turn, arranged with the manufacturer to have the patient visit the shop during lunch hour the next day.

Again, the simple groundwork laid by the business agent had important clinical implications. It permitted the patient to visit the shop in his role as potential worker rather than as patient. Entrance under union auspices became a therapeutic act.

Accepted by boss and co-workers during his visit, the patient returned to work the next day, although still residing in the hospital. After several weeks of successful re-employment, the hospital informed the clinic that the patient was ready for residence in the community and needed a therapy program outside the hospital. Within four weeks of employment, the patient was living in the community, participating in a group therapy program at the clinic, and continuing a successful work readjustment.

Despite the elaborate "game plan," however, only half the hospitalized workers were able to maintain productive employment in the clothing industry after discharge. Some experienced additional hospitalization, a few transferred to other industries and the remaining individuals dropped out of the labor force.

As one reviews the treatment process which unfolded at the Sidney Hillman Health Center, several realities became clear. There was no "typical blue-collar worker," but rather a mix of human beings with different problems, different needs and different ways of responding to treatment. They tended to trust a facility in their world of work and to maintain their treatment relationship when the appropriate modalities were applied. Some were highly verbal, others not, some were responsive to medication, others rejected any "pills."

A second set of conclusions, having to do with the division of labor, also became established. Community facilities proved able to care for these workers, particularly when they were adequately prepared for the referral and the facility maintained ties with the world of work. Labor and management served as significant allies in many dimensions involved not only in vocational rehabilitation but in clinical activity as well. The community mental health movement has as its goal the reaching of people within their communities. The neighborhood and the school, thus far, have been the prime targets of such efforts. It was the experience of this program that the functional community of the world of work may be equally amenable as such a target.

6

Harnessing Existing Union
and Management Resources

In almost any setting where workers interact, there are some within the group who are called upon daily to address themselves to the mental health problems of labor force participants and their dependents. These helping individuals may be formally designated to perform this role or informally sought out by workers in need. Within the men's clothing industry business agents, shop stewards and other union officials as well as foremen, production managers and personnel representatives find themselves enmeshed constantly with emotional problems, many of which interfere with a worker's ability to perform on the job. The foreman who sees a productive morning employee become an afternoon alcoholic can do more than recommend disciplinary action. The shop steward confronted by a union member who fantasizes endless grievances has other alternatives besides ignoring the worker or filing another fruitless complaint. In essence they can do more but often, despite the best intent, feel unable to do so.

The question for the clinic became, "How can these potentials be mobilized in the cause of better care for the emotionally ill?" It will be the purpose of this chapter to report and examine the special efforts that were made to harness the human resources. The intent was to establish a genuine industry-wide approach to mental health care. The two specific projects to be described involve an experimental program with a factory and a collaborative effort with

Amalgamated business agents. Thus, this chapter will concern itself with how a clinic can narrow the gap between professionals and the institutions and constituents of the world of work by developing new ties and marshaling resources in new ways.

The Clothing Factory—A Terrain for Mental Health Care

There has been some interface between mental health professionals and the factory system in which over 20 million Americans spend their workday. Some clinicians have been employed for a period of time at blue-collar jobs. Others are the offspring of parents who spent their lifetime in some manufacturing industry. In general, however, the clinician has had minimal contact with the world of the manual laborer. Gaining access to the factory floor, moving among clothing racks, interviewing on the other side of a steaming iron, delivering services without disrupting production— these are hardly the skills within the reservoir of the well-trained therapist. There was, however, no better place than a clothing factory to explore how day-to-day emotional problems become apparent in the workplace and to examine who and what, within the shop, could be called on to service needs, once identified. The adventuresome and potentially hazardous decision was made, therefore, to enter the alien terrain of a clothing factory.[1] The site selected for this endeavor was the Eastover plant,[2] a manufacturer of medium-priced sports jackets. The labor force consisting of over 100, was evenly divided between men and women who were predominantly Italian, with some representation from the Puerto Rican ethnic group.

The firm is family owned, and the work force is represented by the Amalgamated Clothing Workers of America. In addition to the Italian owners who are active in the business, management consists of a production manager and three foremen. The union is serviced in the factory by two shop stewards who are line workers.

1. See Antonio Blanco and Sheila H. Akabas, "The Factory: Site for Community Mental Health Practice," *American Journal of Orthopsychiatry*, Vol. 38, No. 3, April, 1968, pp. 543–52, for a more complete report on this program.

2. Although the name is fictitious, the description is accurate in all other respects.

Intermittently, business agents, one representing the Local of production workers and the other representing the Cutters' Local, visit the shop to deal with labor-management problems, many of which surround the determination of piece rates, a system of payment applicable to about 70 per cent of the workers.

Employment in the shop is relatively stable. Unlike many garment factories, there had been no layoff for two years prior to our entrance. Recruitment of new workers is carried on mainly through advertisement in Italian-language papers and by word of mouth among the present labor force who bring friends and relatives to fill job openings. The general atmosphere at the plant was informal and relatively paternalistic. Pay was low, with many of the workers earning, through piece rate, an amount equal to the minimum wage which was, at that time, $1.25 per hour.

The basic goal of the mental health program at Eastover was to test how a mental health program could reach out and do case-finding directly within the factory, particularly among Italian and Puerto Rican workers who were low utilizers of the clinic program. We were also interested in exploring ways in which the social system of the factory could be used for engaging people in psychiatric care and the advantages and disadvantages of such an involvement in terms of a rehabilitation approach.

Since the project would be operating within the workplace, it was necessary to gain the commitment of the employer host. The union arranged a meeting on the firm's premises where project, union, and employer representatives jointly explored methods of proceeding. The union's attendance at this meeting legitimated the project in the eyes of management. Management appeared willing to cooperate so that workers suffering from illness or personal troubles might receive all the help possible.

The project proposed initial contact with the workers through the device of a simple multilingual questionnaire (see Appendix C). This would provide an opportunity for the labor force to become acquainted with the social worker during the relatively neutral activity of information gathering. It would seek to identify workers, or members of their immediate families, who suffered from physical or psychiatric problems. In order to avoid the sometimes threatening, often misunderstood, nature of psychiatric illness, it was decided to offer help with a range of medical, emotional and social problems.

The questionnaire was introduced and distributed by management during a luncheon meeting of the total shop. The social worker's diary [3] records the tone of the activity.

A particularly interesting sight was the many groupings the workers had formed, usually in pairs, helping each other fill out the forms. I observed that quite a few weren't able to either read or write and were dictating to the person that was helping them. I began to use my time reaching out to the people who weren't filling out their forms and while talking to a few, I was stopped by individuals as well as a cluster of people who had many diversified questions, some related to the form, others related to needs for service.

The ice had been broken. Of the 100 questionnaires distributed, 94 were returned, with 13 indicating a mental health problem and 14 others noting the existence of a physical disability. The questionnaire proved an excellent way of entering the system. Through it the social worker became visible, his services received sanction from management and labor and a potential caseload had been identified.

The social worker visited the factory at least weekly during lunch hours to provide accessibility, encourage interaction and reach out to those who had indicated that there was some kind of emotional problem. Against a backdrop of wariness, there were some who stepped forth immediately, so painful was their present situation. Interestingly enough, when those in crisis were approached at their place of work, they did not seek confidentiality. The social worker's offer to talk behind clothing bundles was met with amusement. Workers invariably felt free to discuss their problem at the work site, among the "villagers" who already knew of its existence. A diary entry concerning contact with one particular patient indicates:

The lunch hour had ended so I rushed over to Mr. Oliverie and while he was pressing I conducted a brief interview checking out the effects of the medication. . . . I noticed that he seemed more comfortable than in the office and I attributed this to the fact that he

---

3. The social worker on this program was Antonio Blanco.

was talking while working. It was also a unique experience for me, interviewing with steam blowing in my face instead of having to cope with the rays of a desk lamp.

Gaining entry to begin interaction is only the first level of achievement in the rite of passage process. It must be followed by the winning of trust among the population themselves. Approaching patients at work provided a unique way of overcoming initial resistance of individuals. Actual utilization, however, was influenced by the observation of the "villagers" of Eastover of the way in which the social worker went about helping a few early patients. Eventually 32 people reached out for help for themselves or family members for a myriad of social, physical and emotional problems. Thirteen had confirmed emotional disorders. The others needed help with housing, medical care, institutionalization for aged and ill relatives and the like. They came to the mental health program because the clinic had gained a reputation not necessarily for always being successful in helping, but for always caring, listening and trying—and for doing it quickly, in a language they spoke and in terms acceptable to their cultural values. Particularly for a population which does not customarily utilize psychiatric treatment, accessibility encourages exploration and visibility reduces magic. Together they increase engagement and utilization.

The Issue of Agency

A central question which plagued this care program throughout was, "Does the clinician represent management, union or patient?" Each on-site activity, whether at the union, factory or Health Center, creates its own additional strain in terms of whose agent is the helping person and what the goals of the helping process are. During the Eastover experiment the question at issue became, "Is the social worker working for management and if so in terms of what ends?" An interesting situation which arose during the course of the Eastover relationship throws this problem into sharp relief. The social worker, who had gained the trust of the firm's production manager, received an urgent call one day to come to the factory immediately "to help with a crazy worker." Upon arriving at the shop, he was shown a dozen jackets, each spoiled by a slash in the lapel. The clinician was asked to help find the "sick person who had been so destructive."

Since he knew many of the employees, the social worker found himself engaged in a speculative "who could have done it" game. He quickly realized the dilemma of his participation, called the clinic for counsel and was advised to return to the office for a fuller discussion. The clinic team speculated that the slashed jackets might reflect a labor-management dispute rather than an individual psychopathic act. Whatever the etiology of the damaged jackets, the social worker was advised to call the production manager and indicate that he could not participate in the search but that, in the event that a worker was located who might need our services, we would be glad to enter the case at that time. It was felt that the very participation of the clinician in the hunt could undermine worker confidence.

This reluctance to join the posse incurred the wrath of management, who had begun to regard the clinician as their agent. The path, however, proved well chosen the next day when a faulty machine—a pressing iron with a jagged edge—rather than a sick worker or organized sabotage was discovered to be the culprit. And in the process the integrity of the program as the advocate of the patient was maintained. The therapist is always obligated to the patient, but safeguarding the patient's concern is not always in conflict with organizational interest. The challenge becomes one of searching for common ground as one threads one's way through the mixed expectations and demands of the cooperating parties.

The program at Eastover is not easily replicable. Not all managements would be so receptive, even with externally provided resources, as in this project. Not every union would permit services to be dispensed at the factory where its own credit—and therefore credential with its membership—is not distinct. Nevertheless, one generalization rings out as loud and clear as the lunch bell at the factory. If you bring services to where people are, and attend, at least in part, to the needs of the union and management, services will be utilized. The factory is, thus, a site for community mental health practice and a location where unreached populations can be reached.

Indigenous Representatives as Training Participants

As C. Wright Mills has noted, one of the major means of upward mobility for a blue-collar worker is to progress within the union hierarchy.[4] The usual path involves becoming active in a local union, serving as a shop steward, then holding elective office or becoming a full-time paid employee of the union. The men and occasional women who travel this route tend to be sensitive to the needs of their fellow workers. They rise to leadership after years of contributing voluntary nonworking hours in service activities to their organization and their co-workers. Many have acted as union counselors, members of a national cadre of trade unionists who serve as referral liaisons to community health and welfare facilities. The Amalgamated business agents, for the most part, exemplified this historical progression. They had come from the bench, understood the workers, and for many their self-image was tied up in filling a "helping role." Not surprisingly, they were already involved in offering their own brand of mental health services before the onset of the project.

In addition to participating with professionals directly on specific cases, business agents indicated interest in improving their skills so that their intent to help workers in trouble could be realized in actual practice. A workshop, in which they would offer each other mutual aid in seeking to improve their performance of mental health functions *within their roles as business agents,* was established as a vehicle for training.

It actually began in March, 1966, when the co-managers of the New York Joint Board of the Amalgamated Clothing Workers of America called together several representatives of the mental health program with a select group of twelve business agents and their supervisors (trade managers). The top leaders stated their interest in having the business agent serve in dual roles, ". . . not only as somebody to work on industrial problems but at the same time to act as 'industrial doctors.' "[5] The resulting workshop met every other week and included business agents, mental health pro-

---

4. See C. Wright Mills, *The New Men of Power, America's Labor Leaders* (New York: Harcourt Brace, 1948).

5. *Helping Blue Collar Workers in Trouble, op. cit.,* p. 4.

gram personnel and the medical director and social worker of the Health Center. The purpose was to seek ways in which the labor union could be engaged as a full partner in the mental health business of helping emotionally ill workers maintain their employment attachment. The group sessions focused on such questions as: "What kinds of problems are encountered?" What are current coping patterns?" "In what way have these patterns proved useful or inadequate to the help needed?"

The general approach of the actual training enterprise might be visualized as an adaptation of the open classroom model. The end sought was different ways of coping with emotional problems in the world of work by increasing the skills of the individuals and the interrelationships of the personnel and resources of the network, both internally and in relation to community facilities. The training, focused on learning the skills necessary to improve service to working men and women, fell into two general areas:

—*those involved in a personal encounter,* e.g. building trust, identifying problems, working out a clear "contract" around purpose of encounter, helping provide support on the job, each of which is related to the input of the industrial representatives in case finding, diagnosis, referral, treatment and follow-up (referred to in Chapter 5), and

—*those involved in use of resources,* e.g. developing better relationships with, and understanding of, the resources of the clothing industry's Occupational Social Welfare System such as its hospitalization and disability insurance programs and its Health Center facilities, and learning about the network of community mental health and other services.

As the training progressed, several underlying principles became apparent.

1. *People learn through direct experience* (What I hear I forget, what I see I remember, what I do I understand). Thus, training took place around actual cases, and over a period of time, permitting each trainee to try out new ways of working.

2. *People who need each other can train each other.* Thus, each participant, whether mental health professional or indigenous representative from the world of work, was both trainer and trainee.

3. *People* in specific institutional roles *can improve their role*

performance rather than adopt new ones. Thus, helping service the mental health problems of workers was achieved by training union business agents to be a better business agent, rather than attempting to turn each into a new mental health practitioner.

4. Mental illness is unlike any other illness. The myths, superstitions and fears associated with this problem create enormous resistance on the part of industrial parties. Thus, *the content of a training program has to address itself particularly to the behavioral manifestations of the problem,* dealing with psychodynamic information only when relevant.

5. *No curriculum can be projected in advance,* for the content grows out of the interactive process of the training group around their actual experiences dealing with mental health problems. Thus, at any point in time, the group could be found involved in such activities as securing information, struggling with attitudes and feelings that tend to interfere with effective interviewing or exchanging techniques for dealing with different kinds of problems.

At all times group need constituted the lift-off point for fashioning the content of future sessions and for involving others. A previously cited comment by a participant seems relevant:

When I first came in on this project, I was kind of skeptical. How could I tell someone in trouble that he needs help? Suppose I really get a nut who hits me over the head if I tell him to go to a psychiatrist? I was concerned. But it worked out all right. It turned out finding people isn't hard at all, because when a business agent goes into a shop, he knows his people and the way they act—the way they talk when they're well. So you know right away when they're not well, because they're not talking the way they usually do.[6]

One of the trade managers summarized the program as follows:

The project was defined as something to provide better service for our membership, and I think the year-and-a-half since that decision, it's become a dedicated project for those of our boys who were assigned to work on it.

We've been happy to serve. Maybe for selfish reasons on our part—because it's created a much better atmosphere in the shops. We've

---

6. *Ibid.,* p. 6.

been able to help these people who have mental and vocational problems. Maybe we've done more for them than for people who are healthy.[7]

The beginning of the business agent program was a signal that servicing the mentally ill was becoming an important item on the union's agenda. To have been selected for participation in this project was seen as a vote of confidence from the leadership. Business agents interpreted it as a sign that they were likely candidates for upward mobility within the union hierarchy. The desire for increasing their ability to help others, therefore, was reinforced by their own vested career interest.

The mode of communication that this program was promoting was different from the usual autocratic style typical both of so many training groups and of the model within the union itself. The first phase of the workshops, therefore, was devoted to shaking down a technology of mutual training with the clinician playing a role of catalyst or enabler rather than acting as lecturer. This was especially difficult because of the threatening nature of mental illness which aroused considerable anxiety and caused the agents to seek refuge in information.

The discomfort the psychiatric dialogue caused the business agents was sometimes expressed in humorous terms. As the group gathered for the second session, there was a good deal of kidding about their new roles. One of the men, for example, indicated that wherever he went he was now called "Dr. Cronkite"; that several union members had suggested they get together money to buy him a couch and set him up as "Nuts Incorporated." Behind the tone of this kidding it was clear that the agents were very involved in the new project and that word had spread throughout union circles that business agents were formal participants in the mental health program.

One of the first cases discussed was that of a man who appeared to develop, quite suddenly, patterns of aberrant behavior which culminated one morning in his walking off the job. Typically, the business agent had been called in to talk to the worker, but his first contact was fruitless. The agent, at a loss, presented the

---

7. *Ibid.,* p. 4.

problem to the group. People compared how they dealt with such problems. Suggestions spewed forth, among them, "Contact the wife," and another, "I'd threaten him with loss of job." An animated discussion of these and other alternatives ensued. A pattern of mutual help began to emerge as the group, including clinicians, arrived at a consensus. They identified that the most important role for the business agent was to interact with the worker in such a way as to try to convince him that he was an ally. Numerous other cases were reviewed. In the agents' accustomed style of reacting quickly to a situation, a climate of freedom became apparent with each additional problem presented.

The Issue of Agency—Revisited

Although each case discussion was approached around the specific role of the business agent, analysis also provided grist for exploring policy issues. Such an opportunity occurred, for example, at the fourth session when one of the trade managers indicated that a worker had reported being helped by the mental health clinic. The trade manager expressed annoyance at not being informed that the worker was under care. He indicated his belief that the mental health clinic was *responsible for reporting back to the union.* As in the factory, the direct work with union representatives had raised the question "Whose agent is the mental health clinician?" Again the clinic faced the possibility of being co-opted, this time by the union. A lively discussion of the conditions under which information would be shared followed. Initially, there was some sense of abandonment on the part of the agents. They found it difficult to accept how, in a "real" partnership, data could be withheld. The earlier pronouncement of clinicians that material in relation to a specific person would be shared only when the worker-patient signed a release, was now *really* heard.

For their part, the mental health professionals were fascinated by the fact that information they had guarded assiduously was freely broadcast by the worker-patient himself. Again, sharing with the "villagers" proved to be acceptable and even usual behavior. Nonetheless, therapists assumed the role of protecting confidentiality unless written permission to do otherwise was explicitly forthcoming.

It was not an easy discussion. Yet it is fascinating to note that it precipitated movement within the group. It sparked several business agents to initiate requests for help with their own personal and family problems since they had confirmation that our lips were truly sealed. It also served to elevate the workshop's activities from phase one, characterized by a focus on case finding and shaking down of a style of mutual help, to phase two. The new phase moved the group to a higher level in all aspects of the collaborative process. Specifically, agents became less reliant on the authority figures in the group and more comfortable in their own mental health roles. A change in the kind of cases they referred was the most dramatic development. Quiet sufferers joined the already referred, acting-out workers. For all these "workers in need" the union representatives were more willing to risk themselves. They extended their efforts beyond case finding and began to examine their role in helping maintain a worker on the job. The quality of the discussion took on greater honesty as they explored aspects of their own behavior which interfered with servicing the mentally ill.

For years the agents had been faced with mental health problems. The difference now was they could move in on a person in need because they had a path of action along which to travel. Their own greater confidence in dealing with the emotionally ill, and the immediate availability of back-up services of the professional, permitted them to function more effectively as "helping individuals." The case of the ticket sewer, referred to in Chapter 1, represented a typical example of the kind of expanded activity in which agents engaged, and is recorded in the minutes of a workshop session.

The case of Jane Clark was brought up. Nick [the business agent] described his activities. He had been at the plant where her co-workers had indicated they found her actions inexplicable and were not sure they wanted her around since they worried about again having something thrown at them. Nick reported engaging "the brothers and sisters" [8] in a discussion of the "antics" of someone who was chang-

---

8. "Brother and sister" are terms used within the trade union to refer to male and female members, respectively.

ing before their very eyes. He felt that in expressing their fear of her, they had been relieved somewhat and that when he told them she was going for help at the clinic, they indicated a willingness to continue to work by her side. They even agreed to cease the teasing with which they had responded to her provocative and threatening behavior. But the very next day the gains of the discussion had been all but neutralized when Jane appeared at work and mounted a mirror in front of her so that she could see what workers were doing "behind my back." Nick brought this situation to the workshop, stating that he was not sure how to handle it.

A discussion of the mirror opened, for the psychiatrist, an opportunity to examine the nature of paranoia and how one deals with suspicious people. Business agents were encouraged to examine their experiences with suspicious workers and identify how they had won "trust" in other situations. The psychiatrist indicated that when Jane was ready, she would remove the mirror. It was recommended that the business agent help the other workers accept this.

Some weeks later Jane's case was again reported in the minutes:

John [the clinician] indicated that she was in an active treatment program and that she had reported to him, "All the things I thought people were doing to me I now see were in my imagination." Nick jumped in, indicating that he had seen her today and that she was doing very well. The people around her had reported to him that she is behaving differently; that she is smiling, etc. The employer stated that she is no longer getting her work mixed up and he was so happy he offered to make Nick two suits. Nick said that the patient herself realizes what has happened to her, appreciates the work that was done for her, and that he saw her smile for the first time in months. At this point Nick asked, "How about the mirror, doc?" and Bob [the psychiatrist] advised he continue to wait until she takes the mirror down —that she would do this when she was ready.

The attitude of co-workers to the mentally ill was obviously a very important dynamic not only in the Clark case, but in many others as well. During the workshops, business agents developed skills in creating a supportive structure for the worker in trouble which they proceeded to apply in the shop for almost 30 per cent of the worker-patients of the mental health clinic. This mental health component was integrated into their usual functioning as union officials. It did not require new mental health professionals.

The Training Process—An Overview

Group discussion dealt increasingly with business agents' attitudes and feelings in relationship to their instrumental behavior. The group leader, acting as catalyst, sought to promote an emotionally honest climate in which the agents could be exposed to and deal with their fear of any harm which might result to themselves, the mentally ill worker or his co-workers as a result of the behavior of the emotionally disabled. Providing better knowledge of available resources and helping agents improve their ability to be involved in a personal encounter with the disturbed worker addressed the source of this anxiety. But no indigenous leader can be expected to overcome the realistic limitations imposed by the fact that he is not trained to be a therapist. It became clear that the success of the group was due as much to the extent and nature of back-up services as to the content and process of the group experience. Group members helped each other try out new patterns— risk more—but always in collaboration with clinicians who could be counted on for consultation and direct services. Jointly, the representatives of the clinic and the union were able to optimize the benefits of existing resources on behalf of the worker-patients, both within the industrial system and from the community, in a way which neither professionals nor union representatives could have achieved on their own.

It would seem that the consultation and training functions which have been assigned to community mental health facilities could be implemented in the world of work through a program comparable to the one described here. Such a program has the additional advantage of linking the mental health program professional to the world of work. Enlisting representatives of the work community gives all a stake in the care of each patient and in the success of the endeavor in general. Sustained interaction of clinicians and business agents around common tasks can build trust and develop working relationships.

The training program detailed above is different in a number of respects from programs presently extant for training industrial representatives to deal with the emotional problems of the labor force. Two general approaches, from which the projected program draws, can be discerned. The first can be identified as "a sharing of information on both resource availability and psychodynamic content." [9] The most typical example of programs falling into this category are those directed at union counselors who participate in a series of meetings where they have imparted to them the knowledge of experts on such subjects as mental illness. The end product of these sessions is usually the provision to each trainee of a manual with a listing of resources, how to reach them, and guidelines for referral. The assumption behind this model is that bringing in an expert who will tell trainees what to do and when to do it will, in fact, lead to performance of the service endeavor. It is our experience that many referrals do indeed result from this traditional kind of training approach. It is limited, however, in the extent to which it provides the trainee with assistance in evolving a "helping technology" for more complex or recurrent problems than those which can be dealt with by a simple referral. Thus, it tends not to be able to equip industrial representatives to service the range of problems of the emotionally ill with which the Amalgamated business agents dealt.

A second approach is that based on the assumptions of the "human relations school," originally enunciated by Kurt Lewin and Elton Mayo, for the industrial arena. This approach seeks to "decontaminate" a work site from those "toxic" forces which cause emotional illness.[10] The advocates of this view cover the intellectual gamut from those who feel mental health is impossible as

9. See for example, Anne H. Nelson, *The Visible Union in Time of Stress: A Study of the Union Counseling Program of the Community Services Committee of New York City Central Labor Council, AFL-CIO* (Ithaca, New York, Union-University Urban Affairs Program, Metropolitan District Office—New York State School of Industrial & Labor Relations, Cornell University, 1969), and *The ABC's of Community Service,* Communication Workers of America, AFL-CIO (Community Services Department, February, 1967).

10. See, for example, Alan McLean, ed., *To Work is Human: Mental Health in the Business Community* (New York: The Macmillan Company, 1967), and John Poppy, "It's Okay to Cry in the Office," in *Look* magazine, July 9, 1968, pp. 64–76.

long as individuals must perform "alienating jobs" and, therefore, direct their attention to changing job content, to those who feel that mental health can be achieved in the workplace through certain human relations techniques which result in better interpersonal relations.

It is the latter group who have operationalized training programs to reach their end. T-groups and sensitivity training have been offered to many of those occupying positions throughout the management hierarchy. Though less frequently, unions, too, have traveled this path.[11] The assumption here is that group interaction, which strives for emotional honesty, will improve the work milieu. These programs may take place in encampments like Bethel, in retreats, in factories or even union halls.

The use of the group, the striving for honest communication and feedback and role playing, are significant dimensions of the group dynamics approach which the business agent program included. Our approach differed, however, in terms of the nature of the problems around which people came together. Focusing on *specific behavioral difficulties in the workplace* was, we believed, more useful than bringing a group together around the generalized goal of improving interpersonal competency, if rehabilitation of the emotionally ill was to be achieved. A spillover of the mutual training program was that outside the workshop structure, business agents began to use each other as consultants in servicing the mentally ill.

This particular program contributed to the development of a norm which legitimated mental health care as a goal of the union system. A hitherto peripheral activity moved front and center in significance.

---

11. Morris Brand, Shelley Akabas, and Hyman Weiner, "Unions in Psychiatric Care," *Occupational Psychiatry,* Ralph T. Collins, M.D., ed. (Boston: Little, Brown & Company, 1969), pp. 371–79.

Developing Links with the Industry's Health System

Throughout the United States labor and management have devoted extensive attention and resources to providing health care or insuring purchasing power for such care to labor force participants. Within the general arena of Occupational Social Welfare,[1] more dollars are spent on health than on any other aspect of worker need. The insurance route of third-party fiscal benefits has been chosen by most industries. Kolodrubetz reports that, in 1970, contributions by employers and employees for health benefits totaled almost 14 billion dollars.[2] Health care has received considerable attention in direct service as well. This has usually taken the form of management-sponsored medical departments or consumer-sponsored health centers under union or labor-management auspice. Finally, the risk of loss of income resulting from illness has been

---

1. Occupational Social Welfare System has been defined as, ". . . a system of benefits and services, above and beyond wages, directed at social and health needs, provision for which is not legislatively mandated. Entitlement to these benefits and services results from affiliation with a job in a particular company or membership in a particular union, or a dependent relationship to an entitlee." For further discussion see Hyman J. Weiner, *et al., The World of Work and Social Welfare Policy* (Industrial Social Welfare Center, Columbia University School of Social Work, New York City, March, 1971), p. 6.

2. Walter W. Kolodrubetz, "Two Decades of Employee-Benefit Plans, 1950–1970: A Review," *Social Security Bulletin,* Vol. 35, No. 4, April, 1972, p. 13.

covered by a variety of disability benefit programs, some as a matter of state law, others as a result of collective bargaining negotiations. By the test of resource allocation, therefore, health care has received amounts far in excess of its nearest rival Occupational Social Welfare benefit, retirement.

In recent years, a discernible trend in these health systems has been the increasing attention devoted to psychiatric care.[3] The routes provided for treatment of emotional disability have been as varied as those for medical care in general. The Amalgamated program constituted one such path. The roadbed of this particular path was to be built on the integration of the mental health program into the industry and its health care system. The clinic staff recognized that, for a mental health program to survive and grow in an industrial setting, it must not only be perceived as relevant to the industrial parties, but must also capitalize on the fiscal and manpower resources of the industry's health system. The health care program of the clothing industry, through both its insurance arm and the medical services of the Sidney Hillman Health Center, represented extensive possibilities for influencing service to the mentally ill. The Amalgamated Insurance Fund, the carrier for the industry's health insurance, upon hearing of hospitalization or loss of time from work because of emotional disorder, can do more than pay a fiscal benefit. The Health Center physician, on seeing the patient with numerous somatic complaints, can do more than prescribe placebos. It became the objective of the mental health clinic to design and test new delivery systems. The efforts of the program to develop meaningful ties with both these dimensions of the existing health system will be the subject of the present chapter. Also included will be some discussion of two modest attempts to link up with community facilities, namely, the state vocational rehabilitation agency and a public mental hospital.

---

3. Morris Brand, Shelley Akabas, and Hyman Weiner, "Unions in Psychiatric Care," *Occupational Psychiatry,* ed. Ralph T. Collins, M.D. (Boston: Little, Brown & Company, 1969), pp. 371–79.

The Health Center and the Clinic

Limitations in availability of and access to community psychiatric services are problems confronting most working people. The mental health program assumed that this shortage could be mitigated for garment workers by better utilization of the resources already provided in the health system of their work community. It required a special strategy, however, to achieve more deliberate Health Center participation in treating the mentally ill. The plan for involvement was based on a set of assumptions about the ways the Health Center needed the clinic and vice versa. From the point of view of the Health Center's medical group, two needs were identified:

1) with very limited psychiatric time available from its own staff, the medical group needed additional resources to which to refer those in need of treatment, and

2) with difficulty in treating certain patients, the Health Center needed a collaborative program to attend to the emotional problems which were interfering with effective use of physical health care.

The mental health program was equally dependent on the Health Center, for it needed access to medical care for many dimensions of its program. Specifically, it looked to the Health Center staff for:

1) participation in locating cases, providing information about them and carrying out medical diagnostic procedures,

2) enlistment of physicians as partners in the treatment of the mentally ill, particularly for those on a medication regimen, and

3) availability of a resource to which to return patients for follow-up care.

Having identified these interdependencies, the mental health program set out to develop channels for implementation of a partnership arrangement.

The Sidney Hillman Health Center was a consumer-sponsored group practice facility which, like most such arrangements, had built-in provisions for accountability and some control over quality of service. It became clear that the clinic chiefs and the medical director who presided over the monitoring mechanisms were vital allies in evolving a joint program. The director, a pioneer in the development of group medical practice, welcomed the mental health project and legitimated it to his staff. The clinic chiefs became an initial target for collaboration. In addition to their administrative responsibility, each provided some direct patient care. They were encouraged to seek consultation and/or refer patients to the mental health program whenever they deemed that such additional services might be helpful. Each case so referred was seen as an opportunity to make the activities of the clinic visible and to provide assistance to the clinic chiefs in carrying out their roles.

Very early in the game we received, from this source, a group of older adults with chronic psychiatric complaints ranging from organic psychosis to severe, prolonged depression. A few acute patients who required immediate hospitalization were interspersed with this long-term population. Both groups represented difficult patients to service but the clinic viewed them as a bridgehead. Dealing with those whom we could help, and honestly identifying our limitations when we could not be helpful, a base was established upon which clinical interchange could unfold. The receptivity of the clinic chiefs permitted the involvement of other medical personnel. Slowly referrals were encouraged and then used to build relationships with doctors throughout the Center staff. Physicians were invited to psychiatric team meetings when their own patients gave written permission. The intent, throughout, was to provide mental health services as an aid and support to the existing physician-patient relationship rather than to intercede between doctor and patient. As with the business agents, the effort was designed not to make psychotherapists out of the clinic personnel, but to help physicians function better in their own roles in relation to their patients who had emotional problems. Not only did the Health Center become the most important single source of referrals (accounting for 32.6 per cent of the total), but those referred through this channel had a greater tendency to become engaged in the helping process than workers whose potential need was identified by the insurance carrier.

A dialogue began to unfold between therapists and physicians. The mental health program generated increasing interest on the part of the practitioners in examining the clinical issues related to the emotionally ill. A workshop, established for ten selected physicians, resulted, with the enunciated goals of

1) helping the physician become better able to diagnose psychopathology at an earlier point,

2) sharing information with physicians concerning those aspects of the treatment of the emotionally ill which they would undertake,

3) working out ongoing systems of collaborative care between Center and clinic.

The psychiatrist in charge initially adopted the style of lecturer, a teaching form characteristic of most medical continuing education efforts. By the third session the persistent participant demand for pragmatically relevant material caused him to shift gears. From then on the encounter took on a real workshop quality. The issues which appeared to be of greatest interest to the Health Center staff were (1) early recognition of psychotic symptoms, (2) a review of drug therapy including types, uses and side effects, and (3) information on such specific problem areas as physiological changes, aging and suicide.

Discussion often took place around such cases as that of Ben Miller, a fifty-five-year-old cutter who came to the Center with severe lower stomach cramps but refused to permit the doctor to perform a rectal examination. The physician presenting the case described the patient as agitated, hyperactive and very suspicious. He indicated that explaining to the patient the potential seriousness of his malady and the need for the test had little, if any, effect. The psychiatrist, with an eye to helping the patient make better use of the diagnostic consultations for which he had come to the Health Center, sparked a discussion of ways of working, medically, with a paranoid patient. The alternatives ranged from use of medication to enlisting the aid of a family member to win the patient's confidence. The physician was able to take from the workshop a specific approach to try with this very complicated patient.

A particularly significant benefit of the medical seminar was that it created a cadre of physicians with improved knowledge in the use of medication for the emotionally ill. The mental health clinic was enabled, thereby, to refer to the Health Center those patients for whom treatment was restricted to a pharmaceutical approach.

understanding of the company's leadership. As a result the Amal-gamated Insurance Fund functioned, in the fullest sense, as a reser-voir of information, a financial resource and as a potential case finder. Although the combination of coverage in the men's clothing industry is relatively broad in scope when compared with the bene-fits extant in other industrial settings,[4] most American workers are covered by some kind of third-party insurance program. The re-mainder of this section will deal with the way in which the mental health program attempted to work with an insurance company. Examining the carrier-clinic interrelationship can help identify some common concerns which, it is hoped, will be relevant to many other settings.

Retrospective Study of Claimants

Little if anything is known about the "career" of a worker with emotional illness. One of the first steps taken upon establishment of the mental health program, therefore, was to develop a baseline of prior experience. We were interested in ascertaining
—who were the emotionally ill
—what resources and facilities had they turned to for care
—what was the impact of illness on their ability to return to work.
The records of the disability program provided data to identify a population which had, over several prior years, drawn benefits for lost time due to "nervous and mental disorders."[5] These cases had been reported to the predecessor of the mental health program,[6] a physical rehabilitation program which had developed a system of notification with the insurance company. Several researchers carried out a record study of the 131 union members so identified.

---

4. Disability insurance is required by law in only four states, among them New York, and plans outside those states are infrequent, nor do many health insurance policies provide in-patient coverage for psychiatric illness.

5. This study was under the direction of Dr. Sylvia Scribner.

6. Initially, only claims lasting eight weeks were referred. This was sub-sequently reduced to six and then four weeks. This changing disability period can be assumed to have changed the "ill population" collected for this study.

Follow-up interviews were conducted with a random sample of 32 claimants stratified for the variables of hospitalization and return to work. The application of the findings is limited because there is no assurance the study population included all or even a cross section of those individuals who drew disability benefits for emotional illness during the period. Nevertheless, it provides a window into the experience of a fairly large group of patient-workers who lost time because of psychiatric disorder.

From the entire pool identified by the Amalgamated Insurance Fund, all cases in which physicians recorded a specific neuropsychiatric condition as a primary or secondary diagnosis were included except for those with organic etiology. In the vast majority of claims it was found that the report of a nervous or mental disorder was a true condition, not a screen for some other cause of absence from work. In 61 per cent of the claims, for example, almost two out of three, the Fund actually conducted an independent verification check by having a public health nurse visit the patient's home.[7]

Of the 131 claimants, 126 were workers in the industry and five were spouses. Seventy three per cent of those in the study were women. This is one of the most striking findings since slightly more than half the workers in the industry at that time were men. The highly disproportionate representation of women among the psychiatric claimants is not only way out of line with that of the Amalgamated Clothing Workers working population, but with the male-to-female ratio in the population of all chronic nonmental conditions referred by the Amalgamated Insurance Fund to the Rehabilitation Project in the same period of time.[8]

The claimants had approximately the same median age (forty-nine) as the industry's labor force. The largest single ethnic group was Italian (41.2 per cent), followed by 18.3 per cent of Jewish origin and 16.8 per cent Spanish workers.[9]

---

7. In 55 per cent of the cases (those who had medical charts available at the Sidney Hillman Health Center) further verification was provided.

8. For a report of the carrier as a case finder of those in need of physical rehabilitation see Hyman J. Weiner, *et al.*, *Demand for Rehabilitation in a Labor Union Population: Part Two: Action Program* (Sidney Hillman Health Center, New York, 1966), p. 28.

9. Although the number of Italian claimants was approximately propor-

Over one-third of the workers used both their disability and their hospitalization benefits since 35 per cent were treated exclusively, or at some time during their illness, as in-patients. The overwhelming majority (94 per cent) of those utilizing in-patient facilities depended on public (municipal, state and Veterans Administration) arrangements for at least a part of their hospitalization period, confirming treatment patterns reported by Hollingshead and Redlich [10] in relation to the lower socioeconomic classes. Of the 49 hospitalized patients, 42 per cent experienced over 60 days of in-patient care. Those who were hospitalized tended to be most likely to receive the specialized care of a mental health professional. It is also interesting to note that over 50 per cent of the population with emotional disorder had, as a primary treatment source, a general medical practitioner.

During the follow-up study, interview content often touched on the nature of the care provided. The worker who reported, "I once went to a psychiatrist on Park Avenue. When you are very sick you clutch at straws," was not typical. Family or neighborhood doctors, rather, were the preferred port of call. Although they sent some patients off immediately to municipal hospitals, the report of the study states:

Less seriously disturbed patients remained under their neighborhood doctors who most often prescribed a course of shock treatment for individuals with depressions (one-third of the doctors who were primary treatment agents recommended shock but not all of their patients acted on this advice) and tranquilizers and other psychotropic drugs for everyone. Some use was made of barbiturates, and patients tell of receiving tonics, vitamins and injections to "restore appetite and build up strength." Doctors variously prescribed "rest" or "work" as part of the treatment regimen, but this prescription seems to have been honored mainly in the breach as patients substituted other criteria for the crucial decision of whether or not to continue on the job. Some ex-

tional to their representation in the labor force, it is interesting to note that among those who became patients of the mental health program, Jewish workers tended to represent a plurality with those of Italian origin far behind.

10. See August B. Hollingshead and Frederick C. Redlich, *Social Class and Mental Illness* (New York: John Wiley and Sons, Inc., 1958) pp. 253–303.

pressed doubt as to the competence of doctors to judge whether or not they could work. "Work" apparently lies outside the medical domain.[11]

Claimants in this study were out of work because of emotional illness. A search for factors associated with probability of return to work identified little of consequence. Only about half the claimants had ever returned to work and/or were still at work in the industry, at the time of the follow-up interview. The returnees, furthermore, were not distinctive from the nonreturnees on most characteristics. For example, Scribner reports:

The return to work ratio was the same for claimants within the psychotic group as within the neurotic group. Nothing about work status can be predicted on a diagnostic basis alone. This is additional confirmation that work status *at a given time* is not related to the extent of pathology *in and of itself*. [Emphasis in the original.] If one were to select the "sickest" from among the claimants who did not return to work, we would be able to find one "equally sick" who succeeded in becoming re-employed.[12]

Despite the limitations built into this retrospective study, some useful insights resulted. It was clear that claimants tended to be women, but on other demographic characteristics they mirrored the industry's labor force. Their illness was confirmed consistently by record study, visits to homes, and requests for care from the Health Center. Over one-third were treated as in-patients, the overwhelming number in public facilities despite the fact that they had insurance coverage which would have covered treatment costs in most voluntary or private hospitals. The local neighborhood physician played a central role, both as referral agent for the hospitalized and as primary treatment resource for a majority of the others. Proportionately, whatever the treatment source, more men returned to work than women. Otherwise, no particular factor including diagnosis and severity of illness seemed predictive of return to work.

---

11. See Sylvia Scribner, *Amalgamated Insurance Company Psychiatric Claims Study, Part III—The Interviews* (mimeographed paper, Sidney Hillman Health Center, 1965), p. 16.
12. Sylvia Scribner, *op. cit.*, p. 22.

Insurance Claimants—A Prospective View

The findings of this retrospective study suggested that it would be worthwhile to look at the new insurance claimant at the time his benefit payments began and to see what role the mental health team could play in influencing the course of his experiences. The insurance company, therefore, agreed to provide immediate notification on fifty consecutive disability claims which included a diagnosis of some emotional disorder. The design was to reach out to the new claimant, his family and his treating network with an offer of a gamut of services from the mental health program.

This demonstration accepted, as given, the way in which the insurance company operated. The objective was not to replace or change the carrier's relationship with the claimant, but to supplement the existing treatment with which the patient was connected. The additional services offered were to be directed at helping the emotionally ill clothing worker return to work. A view of these claimants confirmed many of the insights of the retrospective study. The populations tended to resemble each other in terms of demographic characteristics and treatment patterns. Contacts by project psychiatrists were well received by general practitioners who, for the most part, were primary treatment sources. They were particularly interested in evaluations and assistance in helping the emotionally disabled worker return to employment. The patients, themselves, were generally more anxious to remain with their family doctor than to accept treatment from the industrially based mental health program. For those workers who were hospitalized, the most fruitful role for the Amalgamated program became backup vocational advice and assistance. The service to these patients, as for those the clinic had hospitalized directly, was one of job protection and of building the bridge from patient to worker status.

After considerable involvement with the carrier, several conclusions emerged. By the time an individual's case is submitted to and processed by a fiscal payment agent, the primary treatment network has usually been firmed up. Entry of a mental health service at that point can improve the quality of care available to the emotionally ill working man and woman. Thus, case finding by the carrier becomes a vehicle for identifying those patients (and treatment networks) which can benefit from consultation service and vocational backup rather than primary care.

This finding becomes significant in light of the recent expansion of psychiatric insurance coverage. As more fiscal arrangements find themselves at the point of identification of patient need, they can become channels of referral to community mental health facilities which, in turn, are organized to provide the consultative services general medical practitioners seem to require. At the same time, those cases which have not been connected with treatment resources can be identified and picked up for direct treatment. These fertile possibilities suggest that the employee benefit of psychiatric care can truly become a rehabilitation mechanism. It is, therefore, both important and worthwhile for insurance and mental health purveyors to struggle, together, with the complicated and sticky issues of confidentiality and fear on the part of the beneficiaries that acceptance of service may endanger fiscal rights.

Linkages with Community Facilities

Thus far we have described the ways in which the mental health project tapped the manpower and fiscal resources of the industry's health system. The care provided to garment workers from their world of work is, obviously, only part of a much larger health system. No mental health venture, even assuming unusually effective relationships within the industry's own health system, could operate at maximum efficiency if maintained in isolation. Utilizing the resources of the community therefore became an essential aspect of the clinic's approach. The question facing the clinic was in what ways could linkages be developed? A two-level approach was devised. The first involved a guarantee of in- and out-patient psychiatric services by contractual agreement with three community voluntary hospitals. This aspect was discussed earlier in Chapter 5. The second focused on attempts to establish ongoing linkages with community agencies concerned with mental health. This effort involved investigation both of how the clinic could use the community facilities and of how an industrial mental health program could be of reciprocal assistance to the community.

Two probes at establishing such relationships will be detailed below.

Public Rehabilitation Agency. In New York State there exists a public agency which provides rehabilitation care including finances for psychiatric treatment. This constituted a potentially valuable resource for securing needed services. Two formidable problems confronted the clinic in capitalizing on the potential. A complicated process for establishing eligibility, which included restrictive definitions of need, was accompanied by lengthy delays in determination, typical of such highly bureaucratized systems. Connecting this valuable but lumbering arrangement with the problems of a fast-moving industry where "time is money" was never completely achieved. From the clinic's point of view, the biggest single problem was getting the Division of Vocational Rehabilitation to accept that a worker tottering on the brink of losing his job was as much a candidate for rehabilitation as the worker who had already severed his employment. Preventive rehabilitation as a concept was slow in being accepted. It required policy discussions at a level higher than the local office which serviced the project.

Neither the traffic nor the problems were all one-way, however. The DVR requested help in securing on-the-job training in the clothing industry for some of its own clients. Accompanied by an offer to finance such a program, the vocational agency's request seemed an ideal opportunity for the mental health project to service the community. The union, however, took the position that no form of training subsidization to an employer would be allowed. The capital investment in establishing garment manufacture is quite small, making it relatively easy to set up a shop. The union saw on-the-job training subsidies as means for employers to train a labor force and run away to nonunion geographic areas. It had adopted, therefore, a national policy of rejecting all government funds for training. No allowance for out-of-industry physically or emotionally disabled could be negotiated. The policies, therefore, of both the public agency and the union were irreconcilable and prevented two organizations with common needs from working together.

The clinic, as a middleman, was able, however, to get some

psychiatric care paid for, particularly for those who were out of work. It was able to enlist the union's cooperation in locating jobs for already trained DVR clients. The full potential for the vocational agency to become a partner in rehabilitation efforts immediately within the world of work—in a variety of industrial settings—remained exciting but still unrealized by the end of the Amalgamated project.

A State Mental Hospital. At the time of the project, the state hospitals, long repositories for those with chronic psychiatric illness, were casting about for new ways of handling their patient population. The movement was expressed in major efforts at hospital release and community maintenance programs. Profoundly needed to help assure success in such efforts were job opportunities for the hospital dischargees and on-site supportive services for those placed in employment. As a demonstration research enterprise, the mental health program sought to identify a variety of patterns of relationship between the industry, its constituent parts, and the community. At the same time the traditions and prevailing sense of social consciousness of the union and the industry were hospitable to developing two-way relationships with the community. All these forces were brought together in an exploratory program between the project and a local state hospital. The objective of the collaboration was to identify the possibilities and the problems encountered in helping hospitalized patients awaiting discharge find and maintain employment.

The hospital selected and referred to the project over 20 candidates whom they deemed ready and able to function as garment workers while they were still hospital patients. The industry, which before the onset of the mental health program probably would not have seriously considered recruits with a history of mental illness, proved receptive to these candidates. The trust which had been built up by clinic personnel within the men's clothing industry and the consequent reduction of discomfort felt by union and management representatives when confronted by the emotionally disturbed, helped open jobs. Very few candidates, however, were able to make the adjustment from the protected institutional environment to the world of active employment. Some were too sick, others had been in the hospital too long, or were ill prepared to understand why they were being sent to the project in the first place. Despite the failure to achieve the work goal for these patients, diagnostic information fed back to the hospital proved valuable. Of the few who were able to return to work through this project, the most successful had been garment workers previously.

A considerable amount of clinical backup services was necessary to assist the few who continued at work. In addition they had to overcome such nitty-gritty problems as having appropriate clothes in which to return to work, carfare and lunch money for interviews and work attendance prior to their first paycheck. They had to work with the frustrations of obtaining release from the hospital early enough in the morning to meet their work schedule as well as facing the problems of securing housing at the point of discharge. Despite the industry's apparent willingness to make jobs available, based on their trust and appreciation of the mental health team's service to their labor force, success was not assured. The transition from the institution to the outside world was a more complicated one than either the project or the hospital had fully appreciated. The value of links between the mental health clinic and the hospital was confirmed by this modest experiment. Confirmed also was the need for these links to be forged with great care and ongoing attention.

In the men's clothing industry, there were existing systems which were involved with, but inadequately addressing, the problems of the emotionally disabled. It became an objective of the mental health clinic to harness these resources of money and manpower in an industry-wide approach to mental illness. In addition, the project sought to link up with the community facilities so that the occupational health system could optimize the care provided to the emotionally ill worker. Some modest efforts were made to pave the street in both directions so that those in the community might benefit from aspects of the industry's health system. Although not all these efforts were resounding successes by any means, they did identify the potential for creative linkages. In the health care crisis with which the nation is confronted today, not all the solutions lie in increasing the amount of resources devoted to new services. If the Amalgamated experience is any measure of conditions as they exist in reality, investment in improved linkages leading to reallocation of existing resources offers an additional viable path.

8

Mental Illness and Work Behavior: A View From Research

From the beginning, this industry-wide approach to mental health treatment offered countless tempting research possibilities. Rarely do those concerned with mental health care have access to specific information about the patient's work environment. The unique labor-management auspices enjoyed by this program presented an unusual opportunity to explore a central question haunting mental health practitioners, namely, "What is the impact of mental illness on an individual's ability to maintain a work role?" Using the objective nature of an earnings record based on piece-rate determinations as a measure of functional performance, a major research effort was undertaken. Its goal was to examine the determinants of earnings in the men's clothing industry and the impact of mental illness on those earnings levels.

The process of this study, and its findings, will be described in the present chapter. Another significant dimension of the research was to offer some insight into the association between clinical activity and continued employment in that the data constituted objective information on the simultaneous occurrence of work and participation in a program of clinical care.

The World of Work as a Research Site

The data potentially available, especially in terms of the population's relationship to the work setting, was rich and diverse. The records of the insurance company charged with coverage of the various benefit programs, the patient files at the Health Center, the membership information from the union and the payroll and personnel material from individual employers all constituted reservoirs of information. The question became, "How do you enlist this network in all its various arms in the research endeavor?"

A special situation for the social researcher is presented by working with the industrial parties. Labor and management tend to behave like secret societies, each jealously guarding a considerable body of information.[1] Given the fact that they operate in a competitive economic order, both are mindful of not supplying data which may be helpful to competing organizations be they other firms or labor unions. In addition, since they face each other as antagonists around a bargaining table, each is loath to share any information which may put it at a disadvantage in relation to the other.[2]

Finally, they often act in alliance to adopt a defensive posture designed not to share with the government any more information than absolutely required. It was the experience of the research team that these conditions obtained in the men's clothing industry and constituted the challenging environment in which research was to be undertaken. The pitfalls were countless—and the project managed to fall into several of them, as will become clear as the description of this research unfolds.

Prior to any investigation of patient experience, baseline information was needed concerning the total labor force. A rather extensive plan for creating a profile of workers was evolved which included two steps:

—a questionnaire designed to gather demographic and work related data was to be distributed to employees in a random sample of factories;

—earnings, absenteeism and tardiness records were to be gathered on these workers from their employers.

1. George Simmel, "The Secret Society," in Kurt H. Wolff, ed., *The Sociology of George Simmel* (New York, Free Press, 1950), pp. 345–76.

2. Hyman J. Weiner, *et al., The World of Work and Social Welfare Policy* (Industrial Social Welfare Center, Columbia University School of Social Work, New York, 1971), p. 30.

Before embarking on the research, negotiations were undertaken with institutional representatives of both labor and management. The commitment of both parties to the study and plan of operation was requested and granted. Based on this green light the questionnaire phase was undertaken directly in the shops and with the active assistance of the business agents. The success of this stage moved the researchers, with high morale, onto the next phase which involved direct access to employer records, the obvious source of information on earnings and such related variables as hours worked, absenteeism, and a host of other objective measures. Without further consultation with the union, therefore, we established contact with the employers and began the task of collecting payroll and time card records. The union heard of our activities. Under threat of terminating not only the research but the treatment aspects of the project they demanded we discontinue in-shop data gathering. It was thus that the reality was sharply defined—sanction general is not sanction specific; sanction from one party is not the same as sanction from both. The secret society reared its head!

The secret society is, however, not completely sealed. The real issue for the researcher is to find the entry crack. A cooling-off period proved salutary and eventually other avenues to the data were jointly developed.[3] The experience of the project from the outset had been that a trade-off was often possible. The secret society gives way when the researcher finds a common ground where the interests of the parties converge. It also provides selective access to information in exchange for services. Initially, the most accessible information came from the Health Center as the sponsor of the clinic itself. Gradually, as sections of the network became involved in program development, the project had been able to work directly with the union which gave us a key to its own "knowledge bank." Even before the earnings study, dues checkoff records had been made available, providing us with a total list of the membership so that we could identify who would

---

3. For a report of a comparable incident which did not have a satisfactory resolution see the discussion of the Navy Yard Fiasco in Delbert C. Miller, "The Impact of Organization and Research Value Structures on Researcher Behavior," Alvin W. Gouldner and S. M. Miller, eds., *Applied Sociology Opportunities and Problems* (New York, Free Press, 1965), pp. 41–44.

appropriately fall into a random sample of the labor force. Our move to the shops had upset this delicate exchange. The raw nerves exposed in relation to the particular research projected were dual—earnings information constitutes highly sensitive data and is, therefore, closely guarded; and further, use of in-shop records supplied directly by the employer was viewed by the union as bypassing its jurisdiction. That the research took place at all is a tribute to the trust which had been developed over the four prior years. Eventually, management and labor were able to agree to making earnings data available from the neutral vantage point of the industry's insurance records. When the dust had settled and the air cleared, the study was, therefore, able to proceed.

Defining the Problem

The reader is undoubtedly aware of the widespread acceptance of the proposition that mental illness interferes with a worker's productivity and even employability. Although rarely supported by substantial empirical evidence, except for extreme cases, such generalizations abound in the literature, finding support in the notions and myths people hold concerning emotional illness. On the other side of the coin, those who have the responsibility for treating and rehabilitating the mentally ill lack definitive information on what constitutes a reasonable expectation of work performance from someone with a confirmed psychiatric diagnosis. John F. Kennedy once remarked, "The great enemy of truth is very often not the lie—deliberate, contrived and dishonest—but the myth—persistent, persuasive and unrealistic." [4] In the case of mental illness, these myths have often resulted in reduced employment opportunities for those with a present case or past history of psychiatric illness.[5]

---

4. John F. Kennedy, 1962, Commencement Address at Yale University, New Haven, Connecticut.

5. See, for example, Charles A. Ferguson, *et al., The Legacy of Neglect, An Appraisal of the Implications of Emotional Disturbances in the Business Environment* (Industrial Mental Health Associates, Fort Worth, 1965), p. 154. They report, "Although studies have shown that employers expressed attitudes toward hiring ex-mental patients that were not nearly so unfavorable as the researchers believed, it is our opinion that employer attitudes were favorable only on the *intellectual level,* not on the underlying emotional level. [Emphasis in the original.] This opinion is partially sup-

The question raised consistently, namely, "What is the effect of mental illness on the ability of a worker to maintain his productivity at his job in the men's and boys' clothing industry in New York City?" was translated into a study built around testing two hypotheses:

Hypothesis I. Diagnostic category will not distinguish between those who continue in employment despite emotional illness and those who do not continue at work.

Hypothesis II: There will be no significant difference between the earnings experience of the mentally ill who remain at work and the earnings experience of their matched peer group doing comparable work.

A complex research analysis was carried out resulting in confirmation of the hypotheses posed. A set of intervening variables which define who a person is, such as age, sex, ethnic group membership or education, proved to be significantly related to job placement and earnings. Mental illness turned out to be one, but only one of the characteristics of a worker which influence his earnings opportunities. Psychiatric diagnosis did not define the work potential of patients in this industry. As a matter of fact, patients, taken as a whole, were able to work at a level almost as productive as their demographic and occupational peers. Differences by diagnosis did appear, however: those with neurotic complaints earned somewhat more than their peers while those with psychotic or psycho-physiologic disorders earned less than their matched group.

For those in the mental health field, the study offers evidence to suggest the importance of evaluating the individual, his strengths, potential and environmental opportunities rather than focusing on diagnostic labels. For present or potential employers of the emotionally ill, and the unions which represent them, the findings suggest that many more productive roles can and, perhaps, should be filled by those with mental illness. The remainder of this chapter will lay out the research design and report and analyze the study findings.

There is a dearth of information on the relationship between

ported by the fact that very little actual hiring of ex-patients was attempted by the employers who responded favorably to hiring ex-mental patients."

illness and earning capacity, in part due to the complexity of the phenomena. The present investigation could not sidestep the complications involved in trying to isolate the relation. If what follows is somewhat heavy and cumbersome, the writers apologize for not having been able to simplify, further, the reporting of the intricacies of this study.

Study Framework

Prior to examining the question of mental illness and its relation to earnings, an investigation of the work and earnings experience of a 5 per cent random sample of the industry's work force was undertaken to provide baseline information. With a response of over 90 per cent of the sample, demographic, work-related and earnings information projectable to the total labor force was thereby established. The analysis of the over 1,200 respondents also established the existence of a "preferred worker" in the industry. Those with certain attributes (e.g. males) proved to receive preferential occupational placement—they received the better jobs. Regardless of where such a preferred worker is in the occupational structure, furthermore, he tends toward higher earnings than his less preferred peers doing comparable work.[6] The existence of the preferred worker had been suspected by the research team. It had been noted, for example, that a cutter born in the United States or Europe was more likely to be welcomed back to work after a severe coronary than his colleague from South America who experiences the same illness. The multiple dimensions of preferential status, however, had not been systematically studied earlier.

The research not only identified the existence of the preferred worker, but defined his characteristics. Once identified, the phenomenon became an underpinning for the study of the relationship between mental illness and earnings. In other words, we sought in our analysis to guard against a finding of lower earnings for the mentally ill which might be attributable to reasons outside pathol-

---

6. See Sheila H. Akabas, *Labor Force Characteristics, Mental Illness and Earnings in the Men's Clothing Industry of New York City,* 1970, an unpublished doctoral dissertation presented to the Faculty of New York University, for a more complete discussion.

ogy. It was necessary, therefore, to match patients with working peers who have the same demographic and work-related characteristics. This was designed in order to avoid having the analysis flounder on the impact of the intervening variables which characterize the preferred worker rather than focus on the mental illness-earnings relationship. Ultimately, the study population of patient-workers was matched with peer groups doing comparable jobs. Patients with the same characteristics as the preferred worker were matched with preferred workers, all other patients being matched with those lacking preferred characteristics.

To guarantee groupings of workers doing comparable work— the conditions necessary for a comparison of earnings—the industry's labor force was divided into five job categories. The clothing industry's use of labor is such, however, that it is almost possible to say that all workers in the industry do comparable work under comparable circumstances. Jobs are, for the most part, semi-skilled. Relatively short periods of training are required and incremental productivity resulting from work experience is minimal. Promotions are almost nonexistent.

The Study Population

The open-door policy of the clinic resulted in 718 individuals being reported to the program as having some kind of a mental health problem. Some of those reported were, for a series of reasons, never contacted by the clinic. Of the 442 patients evaluated and serviced by the project, relatives of workers, retired members and workers themselves who did not have work-connected problems [7] were eliminated from inclusion in this research. The study population—workers whose emotional illness interfered with their functional capacity to work—included 310 individuals. For 17, inadequate records and other problems made it impossible to include them in an analysis.[8] The remaining 293 workers constitute the population of interest for this investigation.

---

7. See page 61 for definition of determination of work-connected problems.

8. Of these, 7 were in managerial positions in the industry and, therefore, the insurance company did not have their earnings records, 7 case records

The appropriateness of the steps taken to match patients with their peers along certain specified characteristics was confirmed by a finding that these patients were significantly different from the baseline population on numerous variables. Having already ascertained differential earnings to preferred workers, the significance of finding differences between patients and the baseline— i.e., labor force—of the industry is that the finding confirms the importance of matching patients with a peer group to carry out a meaningful study of patient earnings. Anything which can be said about the earning capacity of the mentally ill in the industry, therefore, refers only to those who were diagnosed by, and became patients of, the clinic.

Establishing Diagnosis

To speak of psychiatric diagnosis, per se, is to raise difficulties of which the reader is well aware. Making a specific diagnosis is always complex and often elusive. Dunham states:

The problem of validity will continue to plague epidemiological workers in the psychiatric field until more objective criteria are developed for determining psychiatric diagnoses so that dependence does not have to be placed upon the clinical judgments of psychiatrists, which apparently vary from region to region and even from one psychiatric facility to another.[9]

It is well known, for example, that diagnoses tend to stack up in particular clinics, partly because of the self-selective ability of potential patients to choose a clinic which is known to be interested in their problem, but also because clinicians tend to place emotional problems into the molds of their own interests and biases.[10]

In recognition of this problem every effort was made to apply

---

lacked sufficient information to assign the patient to a job category, one patient had not provided sufficient demographic data to match him with his appropriate peer group, another died, and the tape with the earnings record of one patient had been so badly damaged that it could not be read.

9. H. Warren Dunham, "Epidemiology of Psychiatric Disorders as a Contribution to Medical Ecology," *International Journal of Psychiatry,* Vol. 5, No. 2, February, 1968, p. 142.

10. Charles Kadushin, *op. cit.*

a uniform systematic diagnostic procedure to the patient population. In this field where personal judgment is a significant factor in establishing diagnosis, patients of this project were evaluated by board-certified psychiatrists with long years of experience. Furthermore, most judgments were jointly arrived at; the psychiatrist participated in an intake interview with a certified social worker. This collective judgment added to the reliability of the diagnosis. In many cases, supplemental data were available from other physicians, hospitals or mental health clinics and almost always from workplace peers, supervisors and business agents. Patients were then placed into gross categories as defined by the standard nomenclature of the American Psychiatric Association.[11]

TABLE 5

DISTRIBUTION OF PATIENT POPULATION WITH WORK-CONNECTED
PROBLEMS BY PSYCHIATRIC DIAGNOSIS *

| Diagnosis | Patients † | |
	Number (N=293)	%
Organic Brain Syndrome	6	2.0
Psychotic Disorder	103	35.2
Neurotic Disorder	133	45.4
Personality Disorder	22	7.5
Transient Situational Disturbances	14	4.7
Psychophysiologic Disorder	4	1.4
No Specific Diagnosis Available	11	3.8

* According to categories in *Diagnostic and Statistical Manual of Mental Disorders,* 2nd Edition (American Psychiatric Association, Washington, D.C. 1968).
† The percentages in each diagnostic category differ from Table 2 since the former table includes all project patients while Table 5 is concerned only with those with work-connected problems.

11. *Diagnostic and Statistical Manual of Mental Disorders,* 2nd Edition (American Psychiatric Association, Washington, D.C., 1968).

The number of patients placed in each specific category is recorded in Table 5. The most prevalent diagnosis was neurotic disorder, accounting for almost half of the study's subjects. The fact that there are a large number of psychotics (103, or 35 per cent of the patient pool) among the population of patients drawn from the world of work may come as a surprise to some who consider such a diagnosis synonomous with economic dependency. Others in the field of occupational mental health have commented on this phenomenon, well summarized by MacIver:

... the psychiatrist who works in industry comes to view schizophrenia as a more benign condition than his colleague who is hospital-based. Many blue-collar workers who had had one or more schizophrenic decompensations nonetheless do reasonably well on the job. . . .[12]

Nature of Data and Plan for Analysis

Unlike most workers in American industry today, earnings of garment workers continue to be tied to a system of piece rate. Working from a minimum base payment, an employee is paid for what he produces. As undesirable as this must seem to those of us involved in human services, it does nonetheless provide an ideal arrangement for exploring earnings vis-à-vis mental illness. Earnings data were available on a quarterly basis. In formulating the earnings study, we expected that if a change in productivity occurred as a result of mental illness, it would be observable in a comparison of earnings prior to reporting with those at the time of the reporting (i.e., when the worker was referred, or referred himself, to the project), and further, if the goal of maintenance at or return to work had been achieved, this would be apparent by a report of earnings in the quarter after closing. We proposed to collect patients' earnings information for from six quarters prior to reporting, throughout the treatment period, to the quarter after closing. In this way we assumed that we would secure a feel for the patient's earning level before the search for treatment began as

12. John MacIver, "Epidemiology of Mental Illness," *Occupational Psychiatry,* Ralph T. Collins, ed. (Boston: Little Brown and Company, 1969), p. 275.

well as verification of whether or not the patient was, in fact, working after closing.

As the plan for collection of data was formulated, certain limitations became apparent. For some worker-patients, six quarters proved to be an inadequate period over which to observe the prior trend of a patient's earnings, particularly in view of the fluctuations in earnings from seasonal forces in the industry (see Figure 3). On the other hand, a quarter, itself, sometimes proved too long a period in which to pinpoint the impact of illness on earnings. Not only was the three-month period long enough to smooth or hide the immediate impact of emotional crisis, but its length also created difficulties in comparing patients to each other when, for example, reporting or closing occurred early in the quarter for one and late in the quarter for another patient. Finally, one quarter after closing was obviously too short a period to provide evidence of trends in earnings following treatment.

These earnings records were nonetheless an objective measure of the functional capacity to work. A patient was considered to be at work if he had a recorded income of more than $200 in a three-month period. Patients' earnings records were examined in different time periods to analyze whether diagnosis distinguished those who can remain at work from those whose emotional illness makes maintenance of a work role possible—i.e., a test of Hypothesis I.

To test the second hypothesis, that there would be no difference between the earnings of the patient-workers and their peers, the earnings of each patient were analyzed in relation to a matched group of his work peers without confirmed psychiatric diagnosis. The methodology for this step derives from economic theory, according to which the earnings of workers doing comparable work under comparable conditions tend toward equality.[13] This theoretical formulation suggests that any differences found when comparing the earnings of the emotionally ill with those of their peers doing comparable work will be evidence of the relationship between mental illness and earnings. The additional step of matching

13. Richard Perlman, *Labor Theory* (New York: John Wiley and Sons, Inc., 1970), especially pp. 105–23, contains a more extensive discussion of the economic model of competitive wage determination for the interested reader.

FIG. 3
QUARTERLY MEAN EARNINGS FOR
MEN'S CLOTHING INDUSTRY BY CATEGORY

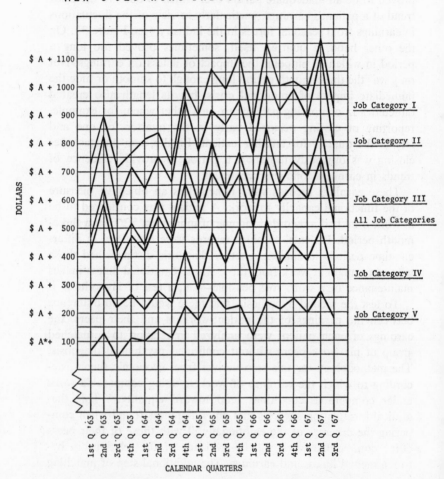

*A is used instead of a dollar sum since the income level
of the workers was regarded as confidential information.

patient-workers to peers with particular characteristics, necessitated by the research findings on the "preferred worker," assured the necessary conditions for the analysis.[14]

Numerous steps were involved in this analysis. For each job category, peer groups were established which provided homogeneity by dividing the study population into eight groupings based on dichotomous divisions along the variables which proved most significant in determining preferred status. Thus, "sex," "place of birth" (native and foreign-born), and "time in industry" (five years or more and less than five years) were utilized for this clustering process. Mean earnings and standard deviations were then calculated on a quarterly basis for each group. At the same time, patients were sorted to identify the appropriate matching group.

The absolute earnings of each patient were compared to the mean earnings for the same quarter for his matched peer group. Using the concept of the normal curve, a determination was made of whether the patient's earnings were

1) above the peer group mean, outside one standard deviation,
2) above the peer group mean, within one standard deviation,
3) exactly equal to the peer group mean,
4) below the peer group mean, within one standard deviation,
5) below the peer group mean, outside one standard deviation.

The analysis was designed to ascertain the productivity of patients who maintained their work role. Earnings were selected as a proxy measure of productivity since most jobs in this industry are performed under a piece-rate system of remuneration. If mental illness had no impact on earnings, category 1 and 5 would each include 16 per cent of the quarters, category 2 and 4 would each account for 34 per cent of the quarters less half the percent of quarters in category 3. If the observed distribution did not parallel the expected, it would suggest that mental illness is associated with an earnings pattern other than the norm.

---

14. Noneconomic forces which cannot logically be associated with differential potential for productivity (and which, therefore, violate the conditions of the economic model), the reader will remember, influenced both the job workers attained and the level of earnings on that job. The theoretical economic model which projects earnings equality for comparable work under comparable conditions, thus, had to be amended in light of the "preferred worker" phenomena to include "comparable workers."

Findings

Work Experience. The vast majority of patients were working in all quarterly periods under consideration. They were referred as workers, accepted for treatment because they were workers and the treatment goal, most often, was to maintain them as workers. Their earnings records confirm their active involvement in the world of work. In the three-month period prior to referral to the clinic, 92.2 per cent of the study population were working. This was so despite the fact that, within three months (less for most), they would be reported as having an emotional problem sufficiently severe so that it interfered with their work performance. This finding is the more impressive in light of a statement of the insurance company which supplied the earnings records. They estimate that due to record keeping and other problems 5 per cent of the labor force normally lacks earnings records in any quarter.[15]

The bottom line of Table 6 shows the proportion of patients who are unable to maintain their work in each time period. Using earnings records as an objective indicator of job maintenance, the reader will note that the proportion of patients who are able to continue at work declines somewhat through the quarter of reporting (87.4 per cent) and the quarter in which treatment is begun (84.2 per cent). The low is reached in the quarter of closing (73.4 per cent), and then the proportion of those working increases sharply in the quarter after termination of treatment (79.9 per cent). The difference between the quarter of closing and the one immediately following closing suggests that there is a group for whom the impact of illness on maintenance of work is extremely transient. The overwhelming finding about work experience of the patients of the mental health-rehabilitation program is that *most of our patients continued at work throughout the observation period.*

---

15. All earnings data were made available by the Amalgamated Insurance Fund. This company is charged with responsibility for payment of all health and welfare benefits under the collective bargaining agreement. In this role it receives payroll data from each employer quarterly. Temporary disengagement from work (layoffs, physical illness and personal choice) as well as record errors account for the 5 per cent estimate.

While this is not offered as a measure of the success of the project, it seems reasonable to conclude that

1) many of those under care for emotional disorder can continue at work;

2) the numbers continuing at work were higher than might otherwise be the case, had the care offered been less concerned with the maintenance of work goal.

Of course, only a control group design, an issue to be discussed later, could verify the latter impression.

Nonetheless, there were 20 per cent not working a quarter after closing. Those whom we helped retire or leave the industry for other employment, as well as hospitalized workers whose cases were closed out, account for some of these. Another 5 per cent are attributable, as noted above, to slow and/or inadequate bookkeeping. There remains, however, a small group, the exact size of which is unknown, who do not maintain themselves at or return to work—a group which fell by the wayside in spite of services available directly in the world of work.

Work Experience, by Diagnosis. Several diagnostic categories include so few patients that findings in relation to them must be read with great caution. Nonetheless, certain patterns emerge as can be seen from Table 6. The percent of those with transitional situational disturbances who have no earnings record is greater than for any other diagnostic category in the quarter prior to reporting. This illness appears to have the earliest impact on work attachment, but these patients return to work rapidly. Organic brain syndromes, as might be expected, have severe impact on ability to remain at work. More than half the workers with this diagnosis were out of the labor force at the time of case closing and thereafter.

Two major diagnostic groups are those with a psychotic disorder and those with a neurotic disorder. The difference in terms of work maintenance is in the predictable direction. In most of the specified periods, the psychotics experienced more disengagement from work than the neurotics. Thus, a smaller proportion of those with psychotic disorders continue working than the average for all diagnoses. Alternatively, more of those with neurotic disorders have recorded earnings in each period under study than the average

Diagnosis	Total number of patients w/diag.	Number with no earnings in quarter prior to reporting	% in diagnostic category with no earnings in quarter	Number with no earnings in quarter of reporting	% in diagnostic category with no earnings in quarter	Number with no earnings in quarter when treatment began	% in diagnostic category with no earnings in quarter	Number with no earnings in quarter of closing	% in diagnostic category with no earnings in quarter	Number with no earnings in quarter after closing	% in diagnostic category with no earnings in quarter
Organic Brain Syndrome	6	—	—	2	33.0	2	33.0	5	83.3	3	50.0
Psychotic Disorder	103	10	9.7	12	11.6	17	16.5	31	30.0	30	29.1
Neurotic Disorder	133	8	6.1	17	12.8	19	14.3	29	21.8	22	16.5
Personality Disorder	22	2	9.1	1	4.5	2	9.1	5	22.7	1	4.5
Trans. Situational Disturbance	14	2	14.3	3	21.4	4	28.6	3	21.4	2	14.3
Psychophysiologic Disorder	4	—	—	—	—	—	—	—	—	—	—
No Specific Diagnosis Available	11	1	9.0	2	18.1	2	18.1	5	45.4	1	9.1
Total All Patients, All Diagnoses	293	23	7.8	37	12.6	46	15.7	78	26.6	59	20.1

for all diagnoses. But one must add that at no time are more than 30 per cent of those patients with mental illness diagnosed as psychosis out of the active labor force. Their ability to maintain themselves as participants in the world of work stands as one of the significant findings of this study. In essence, the data suggest confirmation of Hypothesis I. *The percent of those able to maintain employment is not sufficiently different from one diagnosis to another to warrant the use of diagnosis as a predictor of the continued employability of mentally ill workers in the men's clothing industry.*

Earnings Experience. Patients, when matched with their peer groups, tend to earnings levels which are distributed about the mean in approximately a normal curve. That patient earnings are not significantly different than other workers is the single most important impression which emerges from the analysis. This is particularly impressive when one remembers that most earnings are a result of piece-rate payments. Just coming to the workplace would not, as it would for salaried personnel, keep the mental health patients' earning at peer levels. Those under clinic care had to produce, minute by minute, at a rate equal to their benchmates or their earnings would have fallen below the level of their peers.

Table 7 summarizes this relationship of patient earnings to mean peer group earnings for each diagnostic category. As a matter of fact, those with a diagnosis of neurotic disorder, the largest single group of patients, tend to earn more than their matched peer groups at every point in the frequency distribution. For patients with other diagnoses, however, earnings consistently edge toward the lower side. Once again the reader is reminded that the numbers of patients in several diagnostic categories are so small that the findings in relation to them must be interpreted cautiously.

As might be predicted, those with organic brain disorders experience exceedingly low earnings even if they remain at work. Only 42 per cent of them, against an expected 84 per cent if mental illness was not associated with differential earnings, had recorded earnings of not less than one standard deviation below the mean of their matched peers. Patients with psychosomatic disorders immediately follow those with organic syndromes in low earnings.

DISTRIBUTION OF PATIENT QUARTERLY EARNINGS IN RELATION TO QUARTERLY MEAN EARNINGS OF A MATCHED PEER GROUP, BY DIAGNOSIS: CUMULATIVE PERCENTAGES

Cumulative Percentage Diagnosis	Column 1 % of quarters with patient earnings higher than matched peer group by more than one standard deviation	Column 2 % of quarters with patient earnings higher but within 1 standard deviation of matched peer group + Col. 1	Column 3 % of quarters with patient earnings equal to matched peer group + Cols. 1 & 2	Column 4 % of quarters with patient earnings lower but within standard deviation of matched peer group + Cols. 1-3	Column 5 % of quarters with patient earnings lower than matched peer group by more than one stand. dev. + Cols. 1-4
Expected % if patient quarterly earnings distribution same as matched peer group	16.0	50.0	—	84.0	100.0
Organic Brain Disorder	—	10.5	—	42.1	100.0
Psychotic Disorder	10.8	39.2	39.5	73.6	100.0
Neurotic Disorder	16.9	52.4	53.1	84.5	99.9
Personality Disorder	9.4	42.5	—	78.1	100.0
Transient Situational Disturbance	2.0	41.2	42.2	84.5	100.0
Psychophysiologic Disorder	29.5	36.9	—	66.4	99.7
No Specific Diagnosis Available	2.8	27.0	—	79.8	99.8
All Patients, All Diagnoses	13.0	45.0	45.5	79.4	100.0

These workers with psychophysiological diagnoses never lost a quarter of work (see Table 6). Thus, while they maintained their functional role, their level of performance as objectified by piece-rate earnings was considerably below the average for their matched peers as well as for those with other categories of emotional illness.

For the mental health professional, the data in relation to those with psychotic disorders are perhaps the most interesting. Earlier, it was reported that the vast majority of those with this diagnosis, in this industry, and under the clinical conditions outlined, were able to maintain a work role. Their earning experience, while below the average for all patients and for their matched peers, is none-theless impressive. During almost 11 per cent of the quarters their earnings were one standard deviation *above* mean level for their peers. An additional 29 per cent of all quarters show recorded income for patients with psychotic disorders above that mean. Such work performance from those with a diagnosis of psychosis must, at the very least, give one pause when considering the meaning of diagnosis in determining the extent of disability.

The earnings for those in the remaining diagnostic pools fall between the level achieved by the psychotic group and the income recorded for peers unaffected by the existence of mental illness. What emerges for all, however, is that in this industry, where piece rate is the method of payment, *there is no significant difference between the earnings of the mentally ill who remain at work and the earnings of their matched peer group doing comparable work, confirming Hypothesis II.*

Methodological Limitations

There are certain methodological problems in this study. The orientation of the treatment program was probably not a neutral input in the study results. The clinic expedited the diagnostic process and offered treatment as quickly and intensively as deemed necessary to achieve the rehabilitation goal of maintenance at or return to work. Clinic care and continued employment occurred at the same time. Although associated, we do not suggest a correla-tion between these two events. Yet, we cannot but assume that the clinic had a supportive effect.[16] On the other hand, no claim is made that the work record of these patients is primarily a result of the treatment program. There is no way of telling just what part the clinic played in maintaining the work role. The findings of the study that the mentally ill can work, and work productively, might not be terribly different if the worker-patients had had to find their own treatment opportunities outside the industrial setting.

A control group against which we could have measured the impact of our treatment program might have resolved that issue. No such control group was utilized. Not only would our own staff have objected to withholding treatment from those in need, but, even if a control population could have been identified, its use would have been incomprehensible to labor and management, the program's sponsors.[17]

The nature of the data limited the analytic possibilities. It is possible that ability of the patient-worker population to maintain employment and earnings level would parallel those without mental illness less closely if the unit of analysis were shorter than a quarter of a year as necessitated by the quarterly interval on which earnings information was available. Further, an analysis which would have used statistical measures of significance to compare the earnings of a group of patients with the earnings of a group of matched peers had to be ruled out because of the inadequate number of patients in each cell for such a comparison. The method settled on, of relating each individual patient to a peer group, was the best available solution, but precluded statistical tests of significance.

Finally, the work ethic of the patient population can be assumed to have influenced the study findings. Any observer would be impressed with the intense dedication to work of so many of the

---

16. John J. Sommer, *op. cit.,* pp. 558–63; Hyman J. Weiner, "A Group Approach to Link Community Mental Health with Labor," *Social Work Practice* (New York: Columbia University Press), pp. 178–88.

17. One aspect of the problems of control groups in clinical research has been well described by Dr. Jerome D. Frank, "And you can't really get matched groups—people are too complex. Further, if you want to contrast the results of treatment and no treatment, you have to let one group of patients go without therapy for several months, which is hard to reconcile with one's conscience." From Herbert Yahraes, "How Do Emotionally Sick People Get Better?" *Mental Health Program Reports* (Public Health Service Publication No. 1568, Washington, D.C., 1967), p. 214.

employees in the men's clothing industry. This ethic encouraged patients to maintain themselves at, or return to work, beyond what might be expected to prevail in other sectors of the society. The extent of that influence, however, remains unspecified.

This study sought to examine the work potential and earnings ability of a group of men and women who, because of emotional disorder, have required psychiatric treatment in order to maintain themselves at work. The wealth of data available, and customarily collected by the institutional parties in the world of work, made the study possible. The findings indicate that, at least for this population, the determinants of earnings were a set of intervening variables which identified a "preferred worker" rather than mental illness per se. Although there were some differences by diagnosis, one could say that, regardless of diagnosis, a large portion of the patient-workers were able to work at a level as productive as their demographic and occupational peers. What emerges is that psychiatric diagnoses, established by competent professionals within generally accepted guidelines, do not define the work potential of patients in this industry under the conditions of the setting described herein. It is not suggested that diagnosis is irrelevant but merely that, in the culture of the workplace of the men's clothing industry, *what people suffer from does not tell you what they can do; moreover, what the mental health professionals say they suffer from does not predict how they will function.* If the findings of this study are valid, they suggest that a job may be very much within the ability of someone who is identified as having a confirmed emotional disorder. The productive roles these patient-workers occupied indicate that this is possible and that worksite clinics, such as this project developed, which service an industrial community within the world of work, may constitute one approach to the continued employment of the mentally ill.

Conclusions and Implications

The moment a mental health program leaves the sanctity of its separate existence and moves toward developing a linkage with community—be it a block association, a school, or an industrial setting—accustomed patterns and relationships are disrupted. New actors enter the scene. New definitions of service evolve. New demands must be met. New dilemmas are presented. But new opportunities also emerge. This was, in fact, the experience when a team of professionals undertook the journey toward building a mental health clinic within the functional community of the men's and boys' clothing industry.

Establishing a Valid Approach

In approaching the world of work as an arena for delivery of mental health care, we experienced a bombardment of advice in both the literature and the oral expression of "experts." Opinions seemed to polarize around two themes. One stressed the need for a program that addressed itself to the problems of the organization and its inadequacies as a contributing factor in the emotional disorders of the labor force.[1] The second identified the blue-collar worker as an underserviced population in terms of mental health

---

1. See, for example, Chris Argyris, *Understanding Organizational Behavior* (Homewood, Illinois: The Dorsey Press, Inc., 1960) or Alan Mc-

care [2] and recommended, as the solution to this problem, the creation of additional clinic services for this group. Both polar positions represented the outcome of ideological systems with which we did not find ourselves in complete agreement. The program in the men's clothing industry had to arrive at a rationale which would reflect its own ideological orientation.

Those who stress "organizational mental health" include the human relations school [3] with attention to improved interpersonal communication as the critical variable and the sociology of work specialists who view the present division of labor as a source of alienation. [4] Some in this camp even suggest a linear causal relationship between work and emotional disorder. [5] From this frame of reference a mental health program might involve sensitivity training, managerial consultation and job redesign. Rooting out the organizational toxic agents, as in the public health model, constitutes the remedial process.

It was our view that this formulation failed to discern the differences between mental illness and mental health. While we know what the former is, we do not know, with any certainty, what constitutes mental health. [6] It is very difficult to design a program

---

Lean, ed., *Mental Health and Work Organizations* (Chicago: Rand McNally & Company, 1970).

2. See, for example, Leo Srole, *et al., Mental Health in a Metropolis, The Midtown Manhattan Study,* Vol. 1 (New York: McGraw Hill, 1962).

3. See, for example, Elliot Jacques, *The Culture of the Factory* (London, Tavistock Publications, 1951).

4. See, for example, Robert Blauner, *Alienation and Freedom* (Chicago, The University of Chicago Press, 1964), and Hannah Arendt, *The Human Condition* (Chicago, The University of Chicago Press, 1958), especially pp. 79–174.

5. One researcher claimed, "The evidence presented shows that there are substantial occupational differences of mental health as defined and measured by our indexes. Men in routine production jobs on the average have less satisfactory mental health; those in more skilled and varied types of work have better mental health. Moreover, the findings indicate that the differences of mental health result in large degree from the jobs themselves and their associated conditions quite apart from differences due to the kind of men employed in the different occupations." Arthur Kornhauser, *Mental Health of the Industrial Worker* (New York, John Wiley & Sons, Inc., 1965), p. 78.

6. Abraham Zeleznick, Jack Ondrath and Andrew Silver discuss this issue in "Social Class, Occupation and Mental Illness" in Alan McLean, ed.,

to achieve that which remains undefined. The notion of a linear relationship between a person's work and pathology is, we felt, based largely on ideological rather than empirical grounds. The goals of this option, furthermore, tend to be associated more with management than trade union concerns. The hoped-for outcome of this path of intervention—better morale, improved relationship and thereby increased productivity—could not become the primary goal of a mental health treatment program. Since our primary sponsor was the union, even if we were committed to this idea, its implementation would have been unacceptable to our auspice. Yet there are certain intriguing features of this approach, especially its focus on the nature of the system and its attention to preventive activities.

The second approach, of increasing service availability, seemed more feasible in terms of who our sponsors were and what could actually be accomplished. Yet this orientation had its own limitations. A conventional clinical format often leads to ever-increasing costs and professional staff to meet the demands of the population. We were also concerned with an ideological vantage point which seems to accept, as given, the existing psychotherapeutic technology and where the only new ingredient is a new service population. Such an approach, we believed, could eventually have led to another overcrowded clinic with its waiting list and resulting frustrations. Merely to focus on increasing utilization could result in the development of an isolated program, as estranged from the world of work and its labor force as are most community mental health clinics. Yet, expanding services to the blue-collar worker is surely a legitimate goal.

Our own ideological position was that a given portion of the work force is in emotional trouble, most often etiologically unrelated to any particular set of conditions in the world of work. In

---

op. cit., p. 139: ". . . We do not see mental illness as the opposite of mental health. No study of mental health will tell us how to cure mental illness, nor will the improvement of mental health lead to reduced mental illness, if only by virtue of the fact that the two occur in two different populations. . . . The gravest danger, we feel, in pursuing the study of mental health in industry is this: if people focus on mental health, they can ignore the more serious problem of mental illness."

the absence of a clear understanding of the causal relationship between work and mental illness, we chose, rather, to look at the world of work in terms of its positive implications for the individual with emotional difficulties. True, there were some for whom the work setting was neutral in impact, and even some for whom it exacerbated their emotional problems. For a much larger portion, however, we saw their participation in the world of work as oxygen, sustaining them in the face of emotional disorder. We assumed that the best our program could do was to help workers maintain their productive role. We deduced that, located in the world of work, our unique contribution would be to make full use of the resources of that world in meeting the needs of the mentally ill individual. The target population for this intervention, therefore, became those who were in danger of losing their jobs or had already done so because of mental illness.

The synthesis which evolved was a rehabilitation program which focused simultaneously on the individual and the work system in which he was involved. Every effort was made, through servicing the individual, to influence those institutional arrangements which impinged on the functional community's ability to maintain the mentally ill on the job. In essence, every case was viewed as an opportunity to exert an impact on the system.

This philosophy represented a response to the question "Why a mental health program in an industrial setting?" Two overriding conclusions emerged from the experience of operating a mental health program in the world of work.

1. At any point in time, a portion of the labor force is experiencing difficulty maintaining their employment due to emotional problems, either of a long-term variety or of an acute nature. The survival rate (those who can be maintained at or returned to work) can be increased by stationing mental health professionals in the world of work as the hub of a network which marshals resources within and from the community at large.

2. In order for a clinic to implement such an objective and for professionals to be accepted in the world of work, substantial changes in clinical technology and service delivery systems are needed.

These conclusions resulted from activity during which four specific questions served as the frame of reference for the demonstration, namely:

—How can one locate people in the world of work who are suffering from emotional problems?

—How does one engage and sustain the involvement of blue-collar workers in the treatment process?

—What is the nature of treatment and how is it influenced by being provided within the world of work?

—What should be the division of labor among patient, clinician, "significant representatives" in the world of work and community agencies?

The remainder of this chapter will highlight the findings in relation to these questions and the implications of such findings, particularly in relation to the development of the delivery of mental health services in the work setting. The chapter will close with a discussion of some of the dilemmas to be expected when the professional ventures forth.

Locating the Mentally Ill

Locating people in the industrial setting who are in need of psychiatric treatment is a function of the amount of effort invested in the process. The help-seeking stream is always there, but it reaches flood proportion when stimulated. Developing an ongoing case-finding system is not merely one of spreading the word. An industry, through its various arms, can contribute to the process of finding people in trouble. Training of industrial personnel was, in part, responsible for finding the 718 individuals with emotional problems who were identified to the Mental Health–Rehabilitation Program. Approximately one-third came from the Health Center and the insurance company, with the union and self-referrals comprising the other major sources. Several factors were associated with the continuing flow of cases, no matter what the source, including

—the degree to which going for help is legitimated through actual behavior and communications of union and management;

—the degree to which the helping professional makes himself visible;

—the degree to which help is easily accessible through such mechanisms as a drop-in clinic open during lunch and after work hours and on-site availability; and

—the degree to which the service is perceived as adequate by both locators and potential patients.

Engaging the Worker in Treatment

Identifying someone in need does not assure that he will utilize help. Of the 718 cases located, 442 became recipients of service. For 163 reported individuals, no treatment was offered. Additionally, 113 potential patients refused contact with the project for a variety of reasons including the fact that they had already made other arrangements for treatment. By source of referral, those who became patients came in greatest number from the Health Center and the union. *We concluded that the intervention of a trusted human being (physician or union official), and his ability to transfer trust, was a significant variable accounting for engagement.*

Several other variables seem to be associated with successful engagement. For a portion of blue-collar workers, using help will depend on a therapist who speaks their native language. Twenty-five per cent of the patients in this program required treatment in a language other than English.[7] For others, treatment focused around problems in the work arena enhanced the possibility of engagement. Particularly for the men in this population, work is central to their lives. A number of patients accepted treatment as the only recourse to loss of employment. For them, engagement had an edge of coercion since the union or employer sometimes demanded maintenance in care as the price for continued employ-

---

7. Therapy available in a foreign language is, in fact, an issue with which programs designed for workers must be concerned. Foreign stock, i.e. persons of foreign birth or parentage, comprise 33.6 million Americans. According to the 1970 census, the foreign-born were living mostly in urban areas, 43 per cent of them in the Northeast. New York, with 6 million, leads all states in foreign stock. *General Social and Economic Characteristics: U.S. Summary,* PC(1)-Cl. (Washington, Government Printing Office, 1972), *passim.*

ment. Another basic factor in successful engagement was the location of the clinic at a health center. A clinic which is part of a medical operation is more likely to be acceptable to blue-collar workers than one where they must identify themselves as psychiatric patients.

The Treatment Process and the World of Work

The stereotype of the blue-collar worker–psychiatric patient is one who usually somaticizes his emotional disorder, reaches for concrete help particularly in the form of medication, requires directive treatment and tends to be nonverbal. Although, like all stereotypes, this one contained some truth, it only applied to some of the patients some of the time. This formulation proved most faulty in relation to the communicative nature of the encounter. *The blue-collar worker was usually verbal and expressive, especially through time. He was able to develop a capacity for self-awareness, reflection and insight and often rejected drugs as habit forming. It was our impression, however, that the active, directive therapist was somewhat more successful than those who adopted a relatively passive therapeutic posture.*

Assessment of the patient-in-work proved particularly useful in framing the therapeutic encounter and provided a meaningful arena from which to look at symptoms. The question for the therapist became, "What symptoms interfere with the patients' ability to maintain a work role?" This approach to diagnosis was consistent with the specificity in which worker-patients formulated their presenting problem. Interview instruments which emphasized work behavior around task performance, ability to maintain routine and the nature of interpersonal relationships helped gather data for a functional diagnosis.

Treatment, too, was aimed at functional performance. The orientation was to short-term care. For over 43 per cent of all cases, treatment was completed within three months of their original contact with the clinic. This figure reaches 72 per cent by the end of a six-month period. For over one-quarter of all patients, however, extensive treatment was required even in a mental health program focused on short-term care. Another aspect of the treatment process which is worthy of note is the interview count. There were fewer face-to-face contacts with patients than is typical of a conventional setting. Less than twelve visits proved adequate for four out of every five patients. Enormous activity took place over the telephone and with significant others in the patient's world. *In essence, the professional saw himself as mediator, helping the individual negotiate the work system and helping the work setting change those patterns which proved dysfunctional to the particular worker.* This style required constant vigilance and monitoring to avoid undue attachment to the patient leading to goals beyond the functional objective.

Using the world of work as a site to locate workers and members of their family in trouble results in finding many whose needs cannot be met by a clinic which is oriented to specific work goals. The program assumed responsibility for making a diagnosis and for securing treatment for all those who required care.

Division of Labor

One of the goals of this program was to make maximum use of the resources within the industrial network and from the community at large in the interest of treating the emotionally ill among garment workers and members of their families. Professional dominance of the scene would have minimized the contribution of the industrial network and discouraged community participation. *The guiding principle in the staffing of a case, therefore, was always one of encouraging participation of many, including professional members, union and management personnel and representatives from community facilities and the patient-worker himself. To make this concept operational an open team structure evolved which witnessed the free flow of participants, each making a contribution of his own resources.* Resulting from this structural format were several consequences, including

    —change (dilution) in the relationship of patient and therapist and consequently less dependence on the part of the patient;

    —prevention of the isolation of the clinic by removing the magic of the treatment process;

    —development of a structure which transcended the individual patient and his problem to become a system of providing help in which people were able to contribute based on their *own* roles; [8]

—clarification of a useful backup role for community facilities. This division of labor not only results in expanded roles for professionals and significant others but the process also influences the patient role itself. The patient is not only the object, but often becomes an active participant in helping shape the division of labor and evolving a role for himself.

The magnitude of the contribution of the internal and external networks is apparent in the numbers: one out of every three cases received some service from a community agency; almost one out of every two cases involved union participation and approximately the same situation existed with family input. It was possible for a particular patient to have all three resources mobilized in his behalf.

Perhaps the most important contribution from the community was in the out- and in-patient care provided by the three cooperating hospitals. Any clinic which generates demand it cannot service would be unacceptable in the "time is money" world of industry. It was the backup care available from Mt. Sinai, St. Vincent's and Maimonides Hospitals that allowed the Amalgamated clinic to survive as a rehabilitation program.

Implications

A particular kind of clinic and delivery system emerged from the work of a team of mental health professionals in the men's and boys' clothing industry. The program described here was unique in that it created a new resource to attend to the mental health needs of the labor force in the industry. This book can be viewed as a manual, should this ideal circumstance of total new resources become available to an industry ready to develop its own mental

---

8. The orientation, throughout, was to improve the ability of each individual to function better as he approached mental health problems from his own role, rather than have him formally designated as mental health aide. For example, business agents did not become indigenous mental health professionals, but better business agents.

health program. It is far more probable, however, that expansion of services to workers will depend on initiatives from both community mental health facilities and the industrial parties where the base is more a result of remarshaling existing resources than new investments. There are generalizable aspects of the Amalgamated experience which constitute elements feasible for replication and essential to a system of delivery of mental health services through the world of work. Their application is particularly relevant to community mental health workers who have, too long, been remote from that world. They are based on several underlying assumptions about the nature of the industrial setting, namely:

—each industry can be visualized as a catchment area and is, therefore, an appropriate target for mental health care;

—a clinic, to become an integral part of such a functional catchment (or community) must reach for the vested interest of the parties, e.g. the maintenance of the labor force;

—there already exist help-giving mechanisms within such a catchment (or industry) which can be harnessed for mental health care.

Role for the Community Mental Health Worker. For the community professional to reach into industry, he must, in the tradition of the anthropologist, get to know his "village" and how it deals with the problem of its emotionally disturbed members. On one level, the goal of the search is information. It is necessary to learn who mans the industry, what is the organizational structure and what is the nature of the health and welfare benefits available. The process is a slow, tedious one. Trust, a second goal, though not automatically forthcoming, must be secured if he is to gain the rite of passage. Beginning trust, leading to sanction, is usually the result of the honest, expeditious handling of a few cases of individuals in crisis. Like money in the bank, such service creates the deposits necessary for genuine collaboration.

The mental health worker knows the preliminary stage has been passed when the gatekeepers begin to assign real resources and encourage core personnel to attend to the mental health needs of the labor force participants and members of their families. Then, a new professional stance and different technology is required if the community mental health program is to establish a dynamic relationship with the industrial institution.

The new professional stance *is based on the concept that treatment is as much a contribution of the industrial institution as it is a function of clinical input.* Modesty is the hallmark of the professional who can enlist industrial representatives as genuine partners and not as "mother's little helpers." This new professional stance requires an individual who can mobilize resources and connect people up with institutions and still feel satisfaction from his work; who can offer concrete services and still feel pride in his professional identity; who can function as a consultant and still feel he is a practitioner.

A new professional technology *is necessary at the same time.* As the new professional stance requires a modesty of person, the new professional technology requires a modesty of goals. Changes in the intrapsychic makeup of the individual are sought only in relation to those dimensions which impinge on his functional ability. The clinician, therefore, must be extremely competent and flexible and able to tune in quickly to the patient's problem, how it interlocks with the work world, and what parties can play a significant role in resolution. An important element of the new technology is the diagnostic process itself. A long diagnostic runway would be disastrous to the development of an effective program of mental health care for workers.

Rather than pursuing a "fundamental cause," an ecological approach which seeks to identify the "straw that broke the camel's back" proves useful. Approaching the patient through his role as a worker and assessing the interlock between the work situation and pathology frames and expedites the diagnostic process.[9]

The speedy identification of the problem permits speedy intervention, so necessary if job protection is to result. The treatment process, too, must have a functional outlook. *A helping syndicate can be formed and can divide the labor to the degree that it is minded by the specificity of the problem being addressed.* A man

---

9. As a matter of fact, we developed a plan under which a psychiatrist and social worker carried out a joint intake interview and did an immediate diagnosis. See Appendix A for form utilized.

who has an impulse control problem and ends up attacking a co-worker is helped to develop some insight into what provokes his outburst. At the same time, specific control of impulse in the factory is of central concern to his job protection. A shop steward can be enlisted there as a trusted safety valve to whom the patient can turn as he begins to recognize the onset of rage. What enables the shop steward, the therapist and the patient each to understand the nature of his own participation is the clarity of the contract and the constant shaping of that agreement around specific problems.

There are several other dimensions to clinical technology suitable to the world of work. Many are obvious, and are only reiterated for emphasis. If a job is being held, it is clear that easy and speedy access to care is vital. If a man is at work, the telephone becomes an economical and useful instrument of communication even between patient and therapist. If a clinic has an open door and lengthy hours of operation, a particular therapist cannot always be available to a particular patient. Though individual patients should have an identified therapist (or case coordinator) a modicum of interchangeability among therapists is desirable. Patients derive comfort in knowing that a clinic, not just an individual clinician, is available.

Finally, this clinical technology involves a strategy of interdependence. The professional seeks to promote interaction with industrial representatives as much as possible. The successful clinician becomes accepted as a welcome stranger in the world of work—a stranger who can be called upon for help with problems and can in turn call on labor and management representatives for assistance. Thus a trade-off relationship is fostered. Such a stranger becomes a link between his colleagues in the community mental health facility and his industrial partners.

Role for the Industrial Parties. The other side of the street, namely, the industrial parties, have their own responsibility in promoting new linkages. It is now time for unions, as membership organizations, to become more involved in providing mental health service than is possible if they restrict their role to that of purchasing third-party insurance. It became clear during the Amalgamated program that the union, as a self-help organization with a history of mutual aid, can provide real assistance to workers and their family members experiencing emotional illness. If the mental health field is estranged from the world of work, the representatives of the world of work are equally estranged from the community mental health field. Unions provide, through United Funds and other collection activities, major fiscal support for voluntary agencies. It is appropriate for them to make demands on those facilities to service their membership and to encourage workers to perceive the use of such facilities as an entitlement, not as a charity. Resources assigned to an individual who, by acting as an ombudsman, is able to promote linkages with community facilities would encourage a dialogue between clinicians and representatives of workers. The very placement of mental health concerns on the union's agenda, given the considerable political power wielded by the labor movement in many settings, can serve to move community mental health to a new plane. These roles for the trade union movement can be mirrored by comparable roles for management and its representatives.

A Central Dilemma. In the relatively uncharted terrain of practice in the world of work, a major dilemma emerges. A central issue that any collaborative community mental health program directed at labor force participants must confront revolves around the question "Whose agent is the clinician?" or "How can the professionals serve labor, management and patient and not get co-opted by any?" In the last analysis the professional must address himself simultaneously to the problems of the institutional arrangement and of the individual patient. The solution to the seeming impossibility of that positioning is to be found in focusing on the way in which each needs the other. By concentrating on the nature of the interlock and interdependence, the clinician becomes the agent of all and the agent of none. On the other hand, he is always the advocate of the patient in protecting his confidentiality, and in negotiating with community institutions. Finally, the community mental health professional should never be the advocate of one industrial party vis-à-vis the other.

Walking the thin line among the three parties is a delicate balancing act and can only be maintained if the relationship between the professional and each of the parties is one of trust. One of the important ways that trust develops is through the ability of the professional to keep secrets and under no conditions to share information for which release has not been granted. If ever there was a need for protecting confidentiality it is here where a man's very livelihood is at stake. Paradoxically, the content of confidentiality is often different in the world of work from that experienced in other settings. Those who work side by side, and the manufacturers who direct them, and the union which represents them, often exchange intimate information and observations. Much of an individual's behavior is an open secret and is available when it becomes clinically relevant. An ingathering of information on any worker, because it draws attention to that particular individual, must, nonetheless, be dependent on explicit permission granted by the patient.

Thus, work in the industrial setting requires a reassessment on the part of the professional as to the nature of confidential information. Here, too, the balance is delicate, involving the protection of anonymity while at the same time creating the information base under which it is possible to reach out to institutional representatives in the interest of the patient.

The Pilot Project Approach and Its Outcome

The program at the Amalgamated was a time-limited, externally funded demonstration attempt. It brought together a highly selected and unusually competent staff who, by their own ability and élan, moved a program into operation in a relatively alien world. It was one of the real sorrows of those who worked on the project that the program was never fully institutionalized. Though there were some changes in the way various individuals and units in the union and industry dealt with those with emotional problems, no clinic directed at serving the needs of the mentally ill was maintained.

The Amalgamated experience seemed, actually, to have a greater impact on those organizations and practitioners outside its immediate sphere than internally. This outcome is not too unusual in the case of pilot demonstrations, as has been pointed out by Martin Rein:

The name itself—demonstration-research—is both a confession of despair and a profession of hope. There is despair because the needs and problems are so vast, . . . but there also is hope that goals will be defined, the project might work and research might lead to truth—and that when the right answers are found, rational man will adopt and expand them. . . . In broad sum, the assets of the demonstration project are that it is fashionable, politically attractive, rationally appealing, inexpensive, and not binding.[10]

Rational man did not prevail. The fact that the program worked and worked well for many people did not guarantee its adoption. The leadership had demonstrated considerable anxiety from the beginning. Success did not change this general apprehension. The advantages possible from a permanent program were mitigated, coincidentally, when the industry entered a period of decline at about the same time as the pilot program ended. Resource availability and the interest in maintenance of labor force were severely reduced. Under these circumstances, the untimely death, in 1968, of Dr. Morris Brand, the Medical Director of the Sidney Hillman Health Center and the program's major advocate, dealt a death-blow also to the immediate possibility of formalizing care for the mentally ill in the men's clothing industry. Several changes, however, were institutionalized during the life of the pilot program, and remain to this day, namely:

1. *The availability of professional help increased.*
   A part-time psychiatrist was appointed to the Health Center staff and a core of physicians worked, somewhat differently, with patients with emotional problems.
2. *Existing resources are better utilized.*
   Case-finding communication exists between the insurance company and the Health Center with notification of claimants suffering from emotional illness being made to the Health Center's social worker. Some business agents have adopted new patterns of coping with emotional disorder on the job, and have improved their ability to help a worker in need to become connected with the Health Center. Thus, some in-

---

10. Martin Rein, *Social Policy* (New York, Random House, 1970), pp. 139–40.

digenous resources have been brought to bear on the problem of mental illness. Finally, the insurance company has maintained a modification introduced during the project— i.e., coverage of partial hospitalization for emotional disorder (day or night hospitalization).

3. *Some improvement in linkages have been maintained with selected community facilities.*

New connections with community resources were developed during the life of the project and several of these channels continue to be available to meet the needs of Amalgamated members.

It was on a wider base, perhaps, that the consequences of the pilot demonstration were greatest. Impact in several arenas can be identified:

1. *The World of Work*

The life of this project spanned the mid-1960's, a period when organized labor and some businesses turned their attention to the mental health issue. The very fact that a prestigious union was "in the mental health business" legitimated activity by others. Often the Amalgamated program personnel were called upon as consultants by unions and management to share experiences, contribute know-how and sanction participation.

2. *National Policy*

Project leadership participated in the policy dialogue seeking to widen the definition of catchment area, in relation to care for mental health problems, to include industrial communities.

3. *Rehabilitation for the Mentally Ill*

The project became an advocate of a work-rehabilitation philosophy within the professional mental health community. Papers were presented at several national conferences, lending credence to the position that the emotionally ill could be maintained at work.

One last caveat seems in order. Any effort to replicate part or all the Amalgamated experience will be confronted by a major gap in the information base, namely, cost data. The very nature of a pilot demonstration and its innovative and changing practice make it difficult if not impossible to cost out the services rendered or arrive at a cost-benefit estimate. This problem is magnified in the industrial setting by the issue of how to treat the cost of reallocated resources such as the attention indigenous leadership pays to the mental health issue. In response to these difficulties the Amalgamated program chose not to collect any hard dollar-and-cents evidence. We do maintain, however, that we demonstrated the economy of short-term treatment and produced evidence that earnings need not be lost in the face of mental illness.

Thus, as with any pilot venture, the Amalgamated experience was a mixed bag of assets and liabilities. The accomplishments can be attributed in large part to the freedom, opportunity to innovate, and research possibilities which mark a pilot endeavor. The halo effect of such a program, however, contributes to a greater sense of accomplishment than may actually be the case. The outcome is also watered by the strains between research goals and service goals, between researcher and clinician. Finally, the major financing by an outside auspice, while permitting freedom of inquiry during the demonstration, does not necessarily lead to financial commitment for the subsequent period.

For those who worked on this program *the overriding impression, confirmed by the findings of the earnings study, was that mentally ill individuals can work.* We were constantly amazed by the way in which women and men with severe emotional disorders were able to function on the job. Yet, psychiatric case histories from other settings are replete with many who fall by the wayside. It is our judgment that modest efforts at intervention could influence this tide.

It is hard to imagine, though true, that the United States, as the leading industrialized country in the world, is one of the few which *lacks a work-rehabilitation philosophy.* The presently existing system is one in which a vocational counselor places an individual on a job after the treatment program. What we would advocate is a view which sees the world of work as the context and partner in the rehabilitation process.

Such a view positions the treatment process where people are slipping into the dependency stream rather than fishing them out at the bottom when they have already drowned under the flow of illness and permanent disability.[11] This early detection and preventive approach, coupled with a serious overhaul of professional attitudes and technology, can help end the estrangement between the world of work and the community facilities which claim to service the mentally ill and move them, together, on the road to collaborative activity. It was our privilege to experience the excitement and satisfaction of venturing forth on such a journey. We can only recommend the trip to our fellow professionals and their numerous potential partners in the world of work.

---

11. This kind of universality of services has been well described by Alfred J. Kahn. See, for example, "Perspectives on Access to Social Services," *Social Work,* Vol. 15, no. 2, April 1970, pp. 95–101.

APPENDIXES

APPENDIXES

A. Patient Intake Interview Form *

Date _____

CRN No. _____

I. IDENTIFYING DATA

A. Name_____

B. Address_____

C. Telephone No. _____

D. Social Security number (1-9) _____   E. Local (10-12) _____

F. Emergency contact _____

    G. Address_____

    H. Telephone No. _____   I. Relationship _____

J. Prime source of medical care_____

    K. Address_____

    L. Telephone No. _____   M. If clinic, doctor to contact _____

(Underline the Number of the Appropriate Item in Each Question and Specify When a Line is Provided Next to Item.)

N. SHHC membership (13) (Number) _____

O. Year of birth (14) (15) (Year) _____

P. Sex (16)   1) Male   2) Female   9) No information

Q. Marital status (17)   1) Married   2) Single

    3) Other _____   9) No information

---

* This instrument was precoded for ease in key punching.

R. Ethnic membership (18)   1) Italian   2) Jewish
    3) Puerto Rican   4) Negro   5) Other (specify) _____
    9) No information
S. Where was the patient born? (19)
    1) Northeastern United States (coastal states south to Maryland)

    _____

    2) Rest of United States _____
    3) Puerto Rico _____
    4) Eastern Europe _____
    5) Western Europe _____
    6) Other _____
    9) No information
T. Reason for migration to the United States (if applicable) (20)

    _____
    _____
    _____

U. Age at arrival in the United States (21) (22) (Age) _____
    00 = Born in the United States
    99 = No information
V. Highest grade achieved in school (23)
    0) No formal schooling
    1) Some grammar school (less than 8 years)
    2) Grammar school graduate (or 8 years' equivalent)
    3) Some high school (more than 8 but less than 12 years' equivalent)
    4) High school graduate (12 years' equivalent)
    5) Some college (more than 12 but less than 16 years' equivalent)
    6) College graduate or more (16 or more years' equivalent)
    7) Other _____
    9) No information
W. Main language spoken at home (24)   1) English   2) Italian
    3) Yiddish   4) Spanish   5) Other _____.
    9) No information
X. Is the patient's English adequate for therapy or counseling? (25)
    1) Yes   2) No   3) Unclear   9) No information

II. PATIENT SOURCE OF REPORTING FORM

A. What source reported the patient to the central registry? (26)
    1) Patient (self-referral)   6) SHHC
    2) The project   7) AHI
    3) Management   8) The family
    4) Shop chairman   X) Other _____
    5) Business agent   9) No information

B. Who was the first person who made contact with the patient regarding his problem? (27) (Approached the patient or was approached by the patient)

0) N.A.
1) No one
2) Member of family
3) Fellow worker
4) Friend, other than fellow worker
5) Shop chairman
6) Business agent
7) Immediate supervisor
8) Other member of management
X) SHHC
Y) Other _____
9) No information

C. What was the behavior which led to this contact? (28)
Specify: _____

_____

_____

0) N.A. (including AHI cases)
1) Physical Behavior which upset, *threatened* or caused actual physical harm to self, others, goods in production or plant facilities
2) Verbal or Written Behavior which upset or threatened self, others, goods in production or plant facilities
3) Physical, Verbal or Written Behavior which was nonthreatening but which was considered bizarre
4) Request of Patient in seeking help with personal problems
5) Psychosomatic Ailments
6) Other_____
9) No information

III. DETERMINATION OF "STUDY-DATE"

A. Date of Reporting _____ (to be taken from Central Registry Card)

B. Was patient reported by AHI?
If Yes complete C.   If No skip to D.

C. For AHI cases only (whether working or not at time of interview): What date did the patient stop working which resulted in this report? _____ (This is the patient's "Study-Date.")

D. For cases reported by sources other than AHI:
Was the patient working on date of reporting or within seven calendar days prior to the date of reporting?
If Yes complete 1.   If No skip to 2.

1. What was the reporting date? _____ (This is the patient's "Study-Date.")

2. Did the patient leave work for reasons due to *physical illness?*
   If Yes complete a.　　If No skip to b.
   　　a. What was the Reporting Date? _____
   　　　(This is the patient's "Study-Date.")
   　　b. What was the last day the patient worked? _____
   　　_____ (This is the patient's "Study-Date.")

IV. WORK HISTORY AT "STUDY-DATE"

A. The patient's "Study-Date" is (29) (30) (31) _____
B. What was work status of patient at time of "Study-Date"? (32)
   　0) N.A.
   　1) Working, with *no* difficulty on the job
   　2) Working, with *any* difficulty on the job but *no* danger of
   　　quitting or being fired
   　3) Working, with risk of quitting or being fired
   　4) Not working, but wished to return to work
   　5) Not working, unclear or undecided about return to work
   　6) Not working, sought retirement
   　7) Other _____
   　9) No information
C. Did the patient seek a change in job or industry? (33)
   　0) N.A.
   　1) No; sought no change in job or industry
   　2) Patient is unclear
   　3) Sought change in job but wished to remain in industry
   　4) Sought employment in other industry
   　5) Other _____
   　9) No information
D. Employer at time of "Study-Date" or last day worked immediately
   prior to "Study-Date"
   　E. Name_____
   　F. Address_____
   　G. Immediate supervisor_____
   　H. Shop chairman_____
   　I. Business agent _____
   　J. Job Title (34-35) _____
   　K. Method of payment (36)_____
   　　　1) Piece rate　　2) Hourly rate　　3) Salary
   　　　4) Other　　9) No information
   　L. Job scarcity rating (37) (*to be filled in by the Research De-
   　　partment*) _____
M. Grade of garments manufactured (38) (indicate grade) _____

N. Length of time on the job (39)
    0) N.A.
    1) Less than one month
    2) More than one month but less than six months
    3) More than six months but less than one year
    4) More than one year but less than five years
    5) More than five years but less than ten years
    6) More than ten years
    9) No information

O. Did the patient have any relative working in the shop? (40)
    0) N.A.
    1) Yes _____
    2) No
    3) Unclear
    9) No information

P. Relationship to "Study-Date" employer at the time of interview (41)
    1) Still employed by this employer
    2) Employed by other employer
        Name: _____
    3) Not working
    4) Other _____
    9) No information

Q. If the patient is not now with the employer of the "Study-Date," indicate the reason for departure and underline the appropriate item below:
    Reason for departure (42) _____
    _____
    _____

    0) N.A.   4) Fired without cause
    1) Quit with cause   5) Laid off
    2) Quit without cause   6) Other _____
    3) Fired with cause   9) No information

R. If patient is now with the employer of the "Study-Date," has there been any change in his work status in the intervening period?
    0) N.A.   3) Unclear
    1) No   9) No information
    2) Yes
    Describe: _____
    _____
    _____
    _____
    _____
    _____

V. JOB SATISFACTION

These questions should be posed to the patient as to how he felt on the "Study-Date"

A. How did you feel about going to work in the morning? (43)
    0) N.A.   1) Very good   2) Pretty good   3) Didn't care one way or the other   4) Pretty bad   5) Very bad   9) No information

B. How did you like the work you did? (44)
    0) N.A.   1) Very much   2) Pretty good   3) So-so   4) A little   5) Not at all   9) No information

C. How often did you think about leaving the kind of work you were doing for another type of job? (45)
    0) N.A.   1) Never   2) Once in a while   3) Sometimes   4) Pretty often   5) Very often   9) No information

D. How often did the job make full use of your knowledge of the garment industry? (46)
    0) N.A.   1) All the time   2) Most of the time   3) Only part of the time   4) Almost never   5) Never   9) No information

E. How long would it take for someone to learn your job? (47)
    0) N.A.
    1) Less than one month
    2) More than one month but less than three months
    3) More than three months but less than six months
    4) More than six months but less than one year
    5) More than one year
    9) No information

F. How good were you at your job in comparison to others who do similar work? (48)
    0) N.A.   1) The best   2) Very good   3) Average   4) Poor   5) The worst   9) No information

G. How did you feel about how the work is divided in your shop? (49)
    0) N.A.
    1) Always fair; I had no complaints
    2) Usually fair; I had very few complaints
    3) Sometimes fair and sometimes unfair
    4) Usually unfair; I often had complaints
    5) Always unfair; I constantly had complaints
    9) No information

H. How did you get along with your fellow workers? (50)
    0) N.A.
    1) Very good; some were my close friends
    2) Pretty good; they were nice to work with

    3) Some were nice to work with; others were not
    4) Pretty bad; I stayed by myself
    5) Very bad; I tried to avoid them
    9) No information
I. How did you get along with your foreman (manager)? (51)
    0) N.A.
    1) Very good; he was always fair
    2) Pretty good; he was fair most of the time
    3) I had no feelings one way or the other
    4) Pretty bad; he could be unfair
    5) Very bad; he was always unfair
    9) No information
J. What was your first job? (52-53) _____

_____

K. Was this first job the kind of work you wanted to do perma-
    nently? (54)
    0) N.A.   1) Yes   2) No   3) Unclear   9) No in-
    formation
L. If not, what kind of job did you want to do permanently? (55-56)

_____

_____

VI. PREVIOUS WORK HISTORY

(The following items all pertain to the period from five years prior,
up to and including the patient's "Study-Date." (For example: If the
patient's "Study-Date" is January 1, 1967, the period of interest is from
January 1, 1962 through January 1, 1967.)

A. (*for interviewer's reference*):
    Patient's "Study-Date":

    _____
                    (month)   (day)   (year)
    Prior five year date:

    _____
                    (month)   (day)   (year)
B. How many jobs has the patient held in the past five years?
    (57) _____
C. How many times has the patient been out of work for one month
    or more at one time during the past five years? (58) _____
D. For a total of how many months has the patient been out of work
    during the past five years for any reason? (59-60) _____

VII. PRIOR MEDICAL HISTORY

A. When was the last time the patient saw a doctor? _____

B. List any physical illnesses which the patient is currently experiencing: (61) _____

_____

_____

C. Has any professional ever told the patient he has an "emotional or nervous problem"? (62)

    0) N.A.   1) Yes   2) No   3) Unclear   9) No information

D. If the patient does have prior "emotional or nervous problem," was he hospitalized for it? (63)

    0) N.A.

    1) Yes (indicate source) _____

    2) No

    3) Unclear

    9) No information

E. If the patient has a history and was not hospitalized, was he ever told to go to the hospital? (64)

    0) N.A.

    1) Yes (by whom) _____

    2) No

    3) Unclear

    9) No information

F. If patient has a history and was not hospitalized, what was his major source of psychiatric treatment? (65)

    0) N.A.

    1) None

    2) Sidney Hillman Health Center

    3) Family physician _____

    4) Private psychiatrist _____

    5) Public hospital: psychiatric clinic _____

    6) Priv. or volun. hospital: psych. clinic _____

    7) Non-hospital: psychiatric clinic _____

    8) Other _____

    9) No information

G. Summarize any relevant prior psychiatric history: _____

_____

_____

_____

H. What was the patient's reaction to the project's need to contact outside sources?

(Place a check in appropriate box and obtain pertinent written authorizations on the following pages.)

DEGREE OF AGREEMENT

Source	N.A. (1)	Agreed (2)	Did not agree (3)	No Information (9)
Employer (66)				
Union (67)				
Physician or other medical source (68)				

I. Comments: _____
_____
_____
_____

Social Worker _____
Psychiatrist _____
Date of Interview (69-71) _____

VIII. RELEASE FORMS

Date: _____

I grant permission to the Sidney Hillman Health Center Mental Health Rehabilitation Program to exchange information as needed with:

1) Union Personnel of the New York Joint Board, or other ACWA affiliates

_____
(Patient's signature)

2) Management Personnel of my employers

_____
(Patient's signature)

Date: _____

MENTAL HEALTH REHABILITATION PROGRAM
SIDNEY HILLMAN HEALTH CENTER
16 East 16 Street
New York, New York 10003

Name:_____
Address: _____
Date of birth:_____
Spouse's first name:_____
Mother's maiden name:_____
Father's name: _____
Address at time of admission_____

I hereby authorize the release to the Sidney Hillman Health Center of pertinent information regarding my contact or medical care at:
Attention: _____
Name of Agency or Hospital or M.D._____
Address_____
Period of Service: From _____ To _____
Clinic No. _____

_____
(Patient's signature)

_____
(Witness)

Please send full report as authorized by patient above to Dr. Hyman J. Weiner, Director, Mental Health Rehabilitation Program, Sidney Hillman Health Center at above address. A stamped, self-addressed envelope is enclosed for your convenience.

IX. SYMPTOMATOLOGY

Date: _____

A. Name _____ B. Soc. Sec. No. a(1-9) _____
C. Psychiatrist _____ D. Social Worker _____
E. What is the nature of the problem presented by the patient?
_____
_____
_____
_____

F. What kind of help is the patient asking for? _____

_____
_____
_____

G. "External Precipitating Stress" a(10)
   Areas (specify and indicate relation to work performance):

   _____
   _____
   _____

   Level (select one and underline it):
   1) None
   2) Mild (Such that an average individual could be exposed to it without developing psychiatric symptoms)
   3) Moderate (Such that the average individual might evidence some causal relationship between the symptoms and the precipitating factors of stress)
   4) Severe (Such that the average individual when exposed could be expected to develop psychiatric symptoms)
   5) Indeterminate
   9) No information

H. What has the patient done for his problem prior to being seen by the project? What is the patient's "coping-style" or "coping-pattern"?

   _____
   _____
   _____

I. Using the patient's past history and personality traits, estimate his "Predisposition" to mental illness: a(11)
   0) N.A.
   1) None
   2) Mild (Patient's history reveals mild, transient, emotional upsets)
   3) Moderate (Patient has a personal history of partially incapacitating emotional upsets)
   4) Severe (Patient's history reveals previous overt mental disorder)
   5) Indeterminate
   9) No information

J. What is (or was) the nature of the patient's problem with respect to work? a(12)
   0) None
   1) Task affected
   2) Routine affected

3) Relationship affected
4) Task and routine affected
5) Task and relationship affected
6) Routine and relationship affected
7) Task, routine and relationship affected
8) Other _____
9) No information

Impairment is defined as one or more of the following:
    a) Negative change in production compared with patient's own prior norm
    b) Self-perception of being in danger of quitting
    c) Threatened with firing
    d) Quit or been fired

K. Select the appropriate category of impairment: a(13)
1) Not impaired; no prognosis for impairment in next 30 days
2) Potentially impaired; no impairment now but prognosis for impairment in next 30 days
3) Definitely impaired
4) Other _____
9) No information

X. SYMPTOM CHECK LIST

Patient's Name _____
Social Security No. _____ b(1-9)

Please place one of the following alternatives on *each* of the descriptive categories below:
0) Not applicable
1) Descriptive *but not* responsible for impaired work performance
2) Descriptive *and* responsible for impaired work performance
9) No information

A. Disturbance of Feeling
    b(10)—Depressed feelings
    b(11)—Apprehensive, anxious feelings
    b(12)—Excited, elated feelings
    b(13)—Inferiority feelings
    b(14)—Angry feelings

    b(15)—Suspicious, jealous feelings
    b(16)—Apathy
    b(17)—Inappropriate affect

B. Disturbance of Thought
    b(20)—Morbid fears, obsessions

B. Disturbance of Thought, *cont.*
  b(21)—Disorganized thought or perceptions (delusions, hallucinations, memory loss, bizarre thought, inability to concentrate, distractibility, disorientation, confusion, concrete thinking, etc.)
  b(22)—Over-concern with physical functions and with body

C. Disturbances of Behavior
  b(30)—Withdrawn behavior
  b(31)—Aggressive behavior
  b(32)—Dependent behavior
  b(33)—Drinking problem
  b(34)—Drug dependency
  b(35)—Sexual problem
  b(36)—Other socially unacceptable or illegal behavior
  b(37)—Suicidal thought, threats
  b(38)—Suicidal attempts

D. Disturbances of Social Relationship
  b(40)—With spouse
  b(41)—Other familial (parent-child, siblings, etc.)
  b(42)—Extra-familial

E. Disturbance of School or Work Performance
  b(50)—Reduced work productivity (job, housework, etc.)

  b(51)—Academic under-achievement
  b(52)—Reading problem

F. Disturbances of Physical Function
  b(60)—Tics, habit spasms
  b(61)—Convulsions
  b(62)—Enuresis, soiling
  b(63)—Speech problem
  b(64)—Sleep problem (insomnia, nightmares, etc.)
  b(65)—Eating problem (undereating, overeating, etc.)
  b(66)—Motor impairment (spasticity, flaccidity, slowing, bizarre gait, etc.)
  b(67)—Hyperactivity
  b(68)—Other physical disturbances, suspected of being psychogenic
  b(69)—Other physical disturbances, not suspected of being psychogenic

G. Impaired Physical Growth or Mental Development
  b(70)—

H. Without Above Current Symptoms
  b(71)—

I. Other
  b(72)—
  (specify) _____
  _____

J. Diagnosis a(14-15)
  Classification Number: _____
  Diagnosis: _____
  Manifest by: _____

Category of Psychiatric Diagnosis:
  0) N.A.
  1) No mental health problem
  2) Organic and/or brain damage
  3) Psychophysiologic, autonomic and visceral disorders
  4) Psychotic: involutional reaction
  5) Psychotic: affective reaction
  6) Psychotic: schizophrenic reaction
  7) Psychotic: paranoid reaction
  8) Psychotic: undefined
  9) Psychoneurotic: anxiety reaction
  10) Psychoneurotic: dissociative reaction
  11) Psychoneurotic: conversion reaction
  12) Psychoneurotic: phobic reaction
  13) Psychoneurotic: obsessive-compulsive
  14) Psychoneurotic: depressive reaction
  15) Psychoneurotic: other
  16) Personality disorders
  17) Transient situational personality disorders
  18) Other _____
  99) No information

K. Summary Diagnosis: a(16)
  0) N.A.
  1) No work-connected problem
  2) Work-connected mental health problem
  3) Unclear
  9) No information

XI. TREATMENT PLAN

A. Is the patient being accepted as a work-connected mental health problem?
  If No complete 1
  If Unclear skip to 2
  If Yes skip to 3
  1) What is the disposition of the "Non-Work-Connected" patient? a(17)
      0) N.A.
      1) None
      2) Advice and referral
      3) Other _____
      9) No information
  2) Specify type and method of gathering additional information required to establish patient's status for unclear patient. a(18)

  _____
  _____
  _____

3) a. What is the "Work Goal" for the patient? a(19)
    0) N.A.
    1) Unclear
    2) Maintain at present job
    3) Maintain at work through change in job
    4) Maintain at work through change in industry _____
    5) Return to work in this industry
    6) Return to work in other industry _____
    7) Temporary removal from the labor force
    8) Retirement
    X) Other _____
    9) No information

  b. What is the treatment plan recommended for the patient?
    (Underline each category recommended and specify type and frequency of treatment.)
    0) N.A.
    1) None
    2) Medication: a(20) _____

    3) Psychiatric role: a(21) _____

    4) Social Work role: a(22) _____

    5) Group Therapy: a(23) _____

    6) Hospitalization: a(24) _____

    7) Advice and referral: a(25) _____

    8) Other: a(26) _____

  c. Which are the "significant others" to be involved in the above treatment plan?
    (Underline "significant others" to be involved and specify type and purpose.)
    0) N.A.
    1) None

    2) Family: a(27) _____

_____

_____

    3) Union: a(28) _____

_____

_____

    4) Management: a(29) _____

_____

_____

    5) Other: a(30) _____

B. Was the treatment plan as recommended above discussed with the patient? a(31)

    0) N.A.   1) Yes   2) No   3) Partially

C. What was the patient's response to the treatment plan? a(32)

    0) N.A.

    1) Total acceptance

    2) Partial refusal

    3) Total refusal

    4) Indeterminate

    5) Other _____

If the patient's response is other than total acceptance, what would the Team have to do to help the patient utilize the services offered?

B. Breakdown of Treatment Process Data

TABLE B-1

FACE-TO-FACE INTERVIEWS OF UNION MEMBER-PATIENTS BY DIAGNOSIS *

Number of Face-to-Face Contacts / Diagnosis	% of All Patients	% of All with Psychotic Disorder	% of All with Psychoneurotic Disorder	% of All with Psycho-Physiologic Disorder	% of All with Organic Brain Damage	% of All with Personality Disorder	% of All with Transient Situational Disorder	% of All with Other Diagnoses
1–4	57.4	50.6	56.5	40.0	70.00	63.3	91.7	81.8
5–8	11.8	13.0	13.0	40.0	10.00	9.9	—	—
9–12	10.1	9.7	12.3	—	—	6.6	—	—
13–20	8.3	9.1	8.4	—	20.00	9.9	—	13.6
21 and over	12.4	17.5	9.7	20.0	—	9.9	8.3	4.5
TOTALS	100.0	99.9	99.9	100.0	100.00	100.0	100.0	99.9

* N=387

TABLE B-2

LENGTH OF TREATMENT,
CUMULATIVE PERCENTAGE BY DIAGNOSIS

Diagnosis Length of Treatment	% of All with Psychotic Disorder	% of All with Psycho-neurotic Disorder	% of All with Psycho-Physiologic Disorder	% of All with Personal-ity Disorder	% of All with Transient Situational Disorder	% of All with Other Di-agnoses
less than 3 mo.	27.4	42.9	25.0	46.6	85.0	65.0
3 mo. or more but less than 6	52.7	72.8	50.0	73.2	100.0	90.0
6 mo. or more but less than 12	74.6	91.6	100.0	86.5	—	95.0
1 yr. or more	99.9	99.9	—	99.8	—	100.0

* N=387

TABLE B-3

TYPE OF INVOLVEMENT OF "SIGNIFICANT OTHERS" *

Population Type of Involvement of "Significant Others"	% of All Pa-tients with such Involve-ment	% of Pa-tients with Psychotic Disorder with such Involvement	% of Pa-tients with Neurotic Disorder with such Involvement
Family	43	56	33
Union	37	44	26
Management	11	16	7
Sidney Hillman Health Center	15	18	12
Outside Community Facility	33	47	19

* N=350

C. Eastover Questionnaire *

(Rehabilitation–Mental Health Program
Eastover Factory
Joint Board of Shirt, Leisurewear, ACWA)

Union Local No. _____

Home Address _____   Telephone No. _____

PLEASE LIST BELOW THE NAME, AGE AND SEX OF RELA-
TIVES LIVING AT HOME WITH YOU:

Name	Relationship to You (wife, mother, son, etc.)	Age	*Check One:* Male	Female
1. (Your own name)	_____	____	( )	( )
2. _____	_____	____	( )	( )
3. _____	_____	____	( )	( )
4. _____	_____	____	( )	( )
5. _____	_____	____	( )	( )
6. _____	_____	____	( )	( )

DO YOU OR ANYONE LIVING AT HOME HAVE:	Yes	No	If Yes, Who?	What?
1. Trouble seeing even when wearing glasses?	( )	( )	_____	
2. Trouble walking or climbing stairs?	( )	( )	_____	
3. A problem with nerves, worries or a mental condition?	( )	( )	_____	_____
4. A heart condition?	( )	( )	_____	
5. A problem with children or teenagers?	( )	( )	_____	_____
6. Any other condition or problem that interferes with working, doing the housework, going to school or other activities?	( )	( )	_____	_____

Use this space if you need to explain:

Thank You

* This form was also distributed in Italian and Spanish.

Reports and Publications Resulting From the Mental Health Program

"A Union Fights Mental Illness." *Industrial Bulletin*, Albany, N.Y., October 1964, pp. 2–6.

Akabas, Sheila H., *Labor Force Characteristics, Mental Illness and Earnings in the Men's Clothing Industry of New York City, 1970* (an unpublished doctoral dissertation submitted to New York University, 1970). Abstracted in *Dissertation Abstracts*, Vol. 31, No. 11, Ann Arbor, Mich., p. 5609-A.

Akabas, Shelley, "Mental Health: A Report on Labor, Management, and Carrier Cooperation." *Pension and Welfare News*, Vol. 3, No. 9, June 1967, pp. 49–52.

Akabas, Shelley, and Weiner, Hyman J., "The Blue-Collar Worker and Psychiatry: A New Alliance." *Rehabilitation Record*, Vol. 10, No. 4, July-August 1969, pp. 8–11.

Blanco, Antonio, and Akabas, Sheila H., "The Factory: Site for Community Mental Health Practice." *American Journal of Orthopsychiatry*, Vol. 38, No. 3, April 1968, pp. 543–552.

Brand, Morris; Akabas, Shelley; and Weiner, Hyman J., "Unions in Psychiatric Care," in *Occupational Psychiatry*, ed. Ralph T. Collins, M.D. Little, Brown & Company, Boston, 1969, pp. 371–379.

Esterowitz, Ruth, "The Social Worker in a Labour Rehabilitation Programme," in *Basic Services and Equipment for Rehabilitation Centers*. United Nations Department of Economic & Social Affairs, New York, 1967.

Helping Blue-Collar Workers in Trouble: A Report of a Labor Mental Health Conference. Sidney Hillman Health Center of New York, New York, 1967.

"Mental Rehabilitation by Union Suits Its Members." *Medical World News*, Vol. 7, No. 33, September 9, 1966, p. 82.

"Pioneering Mental Health Project Aids Hundreds in Clothing Union." *AFL-CIO News,* Vol. XV, No. 24, June 13, 1970, p. 8.

Sommer, John J., "Labor and Management: New Roles in Mental Health." *American Journal of Orthopsychiatry,* Vol. XXXV, No. 3, April 1965, pp. 558–563.

Sommer, John J., "Work as a Therapeutic Goal: Union-Management Clinical Contributions to a Mental Health Program." *Mental Hygiene,* Vol. 53, No. 2, April 1969, pp. 263–268.

Weiner, Hyman J., "A Group Approach to Link Community Mental Health with Labor," in *Social Work Practice.* Columbia University Press, New York, 1967, pp. 178–188.

Weiner, Hyman J., and Brand, Morris S., "Involving a Labor Union in the Rehabilitation of the Mentally Ill." *American Journal of Orthopsychiatry,* Vol. XXXV, No. 3, April 1965, pp. 598–600.

Weiner, Hyman J., "Labor-Management Relations and Mental Health," in *To Work Is Human: Mental Health & the Business Community,* ed. Alan McLean. The Macmillan Company, New York, 1967, pp. 193–202.

Wittenberg, Clarissa, "A Labor Union Mental Health Program," in *Mental Health Program Reports—3.* National Institute of Mental Health, Chevy Chase, Md. January 1969, pp. 211–227.

Index

183